The Doctor Medicine Couldn't Kill

Kennan Taylor's Journey in Medical Practice and Beyond
In Dialogue with Ian Cook

Kennan Taylor, MD

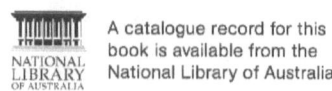 A catalogue record for this book is available from the National Library of Australia

Kennan Taylor asserts the moral right to be identified as the author of this work. Except as provided by Australian law, no part of this book may be reproduced without permission in writing from the author.

Copyright © 2023 Kennan E. Taylor
ISBN-13: 978-1-922727-97-8

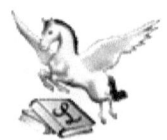

Linellen Press
265 Boomerang Road
Oldbury, Western Australia
www.linellenpress.com.au

Traditionally, a new physician swears the Hippocratic Oath upon a number of healing gods, that he will uphold a number of professional ethical standards.

In the Oath, the physician pledges to prescribe only beneficial treatments, according to his abilities and judgment; to refrain from causing harm or hurt; and to live an exemplary personal and professional life.

Dr Ian Cook died in 2021, prior to the completion of this record of his meetings and exchanges with Dr Taylor.

Dr Taylor has chosen to continue with their various exchanges as a dialogue, with some integrative reconstruction of the period 2021-22.

This approach is a literary device to represent the wide-ranging discussions that occurred between them over many years of their professional and personal association, and remains true to the spirit of our friendship.

A statement to Dr Cook's beliefs and honouring of his life and work, in love; this book is dedicated to him.

It is the considered opinion of the author(s) that veracity is essential, even though popular and legal convention might have it otherwise.

All facts and other accounts in this book are authentic from the first-person perspective. No claim is made to an absolute third-person veracity.

Names and sometimes locations have been changed and disguised, if considered by the authors that such overt veracity could be a means to thwart the intention or purpose of this work.

Preface

Maybe we should entitle this an 'Anti-Preface'; as it is somewhat sacrilegious.

We do not thank the modern medical profession for losing its way with an almost exclusively scientific and technological approach in what was formerly and principally an art. We believe this represents a disconnection from the core principles of medicine as espoused in all medical systems of practice, but currently eschewed in modern western medicine. We are dismayed when other medical systems, both from other cultures and alternatives within our own, are not only ignored but treated with disrespect and even denigrated.

We consider that the recipient of medical care – the patient – has become lost in this process and become a dehumanised statistic, when his or her beliefs and values are to be fundamentally respected. Further, he or she should be the centre of the profession's attention. To present the public with a fear-based and pathologically-driven version of what is a sacred art simply amplifies discontent, as well as exacerbating any physical or mental dis-ease for which relief is being sought. We lament that the social and cultural dimensions remain ignored, despite adequate recognition of their place in health and wellbeing, both individual and collective.

That the legal profession has undue influence in medical management in the West has become a truism. That it affects the decisions of individual health professionals in their management of their patients, over and above their wishes and demands, is not fully recognised. That the political powers that be have created structures that drive individual practitioner's decisions into a protocol-oriented statistical and technological abyss is lamentable, and that the mainstream media largely falls into line with this position is more than disappointing.

We reserve our major concern and criticism for two sectors: that big business and particularly the pharmaceutical industry, backed by the pathology industry, now drive political agendas is now a truism; that the excesses of capitalism and the avarice of some entitled individuals is honoured to the detriment of the health of others, society and even nations, is deplorable. More subtly still, the dominance and control of our near-obsolete monotheistic religious organisations cannot escape scathing criticism for ignoring the pain of their charges, even adding to it, as well as their acquiescence and complicity to forces of power and control in all sectors of health and wellbeing.

We are awed by the resilience of individual sufferers in the wake of everything expressed herein and applaud your continued search for answers to questions often ignored or disrespected. That the physical body and mind are able to endure and transition these conflicting forces is homage to the human spirit. May it long endure, because its voice is and will be further and forever heard.

Introduction

Kennan Taylor

I am attracted to death. At least I think I must be.

The ocean has rejected me after two serious challenges and I have walked away from three car accidents when the vehicle died. After my marriage ended, my broken heart allowed me an up-to-date experience of how the profession manages so-called heart disease – basically, it doesn't very well at all. Add my two serious near-death challenges with infectious disease, plus my proclivity for alcohol, and you'd think I was a cat now running out of lives. Even my orgasms feel more like dying these days; they're unlikely to be about further procreation. Maybe it's all in my stars, like my astrologer friends tell me, maybe it's my destiny.

And also, maybe that's why I was originally attracted to medicine, but didn't realise it at the time. Medicine fears death. It need not, but it does. It certainly spends enormous emotional and financial resources keeping people alive beyond their allotted time. Could I have been attracted to medicine to deal with my own death wish, then symbolically died by leaving the profession, because it didn't satisfy my wish?

In so many ways medicine is a death cult. It certainly doesn't deal with birth and sex as intensely, although it should interfere less with the former and attend to the latter much more than it does. But then again, we have a religion that is a death cult, stopping at the crucifixion and not embracing the resurrection. We need to get beyond death if medicine is to survive; somewhat paradoxically, to survive it must die, decompose and resurrect. Paradigm shift is the polite term for this process, I am told. As I go through my own resurrection, I now see this.

My attraction to tradition has been my salvation, along with new-age dalliances and some immersion in alternative medicine. I don't want to die; I want to transform. But to transform I must die, at least symbolically, and with a necessary sacrifice. When I don't see that the dying is symbolic, it may become literal; maybe I am trying to tell medicine this simple truth of not confusing the two.

Medicine must also get rid of the shackles of science as a neo-religious 'scientism' and reconnect with its spiritual roots, which is there even in our Christian heritage: Jesus the medicine man, I like that. It is crowding in on us from the East with Buddhism, Taoism, and more. It is emerging from our Pagan Traditions, northern and western. Because the doctor is also – or should be – a priest and a healer, not just a scribe or technician. Medicine needs to reconnect to its heart.

Medicine must listen to the people, the public it claims to serve, but whom it rejects in the self-serving of its vested interests; because people are frightened. Yet more deeply, they are tired and disillusioned of a medicine that no longer serves and instead enslaves them. They are tired and disbelieving of a media that supports an establishment position and doesn't partake in its change. They are tired of medicine becoming a progressive tool of a political and economic system that is itself dying.

This is now most obvious on the internet, where social media – for all its shortcomings – is screaming in pain, with dissatisfaction and disillusionment.

The noise is intense. But is medicine listening?

I am listening… I fucking had to, otherwise I'd be dead.

But I'm still alive, I'm Kennan Taylor – I'm the doctor medicine couldn't kill.

Prologue

Ian Cook

This is the story about a man who qualified as a doctor of medicine and then chose clinical medical practice as a career. He had assumed this career would be a lifetime choice, but it didn't turn out that way. It is an account of the interviews I had with this man, Kennan Taylor, over several years and for differing reasons.

I am an academic who works as a teacher, mentor and author. I had heard of Kennan's difficulties with the medical profession independently, so when he engaged me semi-professionally at a crisis point in his career, I knew I would have a challenge on my hands.

Just as I was getting to know him, Kennan made an abrupt decision to leave medical practice, resign his registration, and to operate independently of the institutional health system. At this point, our relationship changed and he then asked me to help tell his story, rather than continue with a joint writing project we had planned to undertake about revisioning medicine and the changes it must then undertake, which I now believe we never will; instead, they may well become embedded in this account.

The meetings started with me wanting to document his career, decisions and their consequences through his stories, together with any conclusions we would come to. Then the discussions became far broader and applicable to other doctors, their patients, the public at large, and the medical profession... if it is prepared to listen. But I don't think it is. Hence this book, and its challenges to the health establishment, as well as your own health choices.

As Kennan's story grew, I decided to write it as a book, the one in your hands, because I have written books – I am a writer and author in several areas, including modern medicine. I felt qualified to undertake this task and turn Kennan's very verbal, complex and journalistic style into an account that readers could understand and also relate to.

Kennan's stories and their meaning are his own. And it is the significance of these stories within his own personal narrative that is paramount in this account. I wanted to preserve this, so I have kept myself and my experience relatively out of the picture. I asked Kennan to write the introductory prologue only and, with insistence, he provided a postscript. These pieces also show a side to his character that is not readily apparent in the main text.

I wanted something personal that would reach out to people, even if his views are sometimes controversial, emotionally and intellectually challenging, even spiritually driven. I wanted to create an atmosphere that we could all maybe relate to, even if it was spartan, brutal, and disturbingly revealing at times.

But I also wanted my readers to get into Kennan's head and see his account – and medicine – from the inside. I wanted them to get the relevance, significance, and even meaning, both to him and for themselves. After this, I let the tape run, so to speak; unplugged and in Kennan's wording, "unmuzzled". I simply edited what I had, then I accumulated it into a readable account.

I also wanted to point out that the stories are recounted with no embellishment or alteration on my part; I can't comment as to whether this is the case with Kennan, though he assured me they are as he recalled them, and … "undoctored"! However, the truth resides in the core of them, and the wisdom is in the account, often left metaphoric. This is to preserve the integrity of the accounts, rather than personal or professional reputation; it is also to engage the reader in an imaginative manner, as in a fictional work. The success of this method and various techniques are for the reader to judge.

Then a hiatus arrived. This work was resourced and initially written in a period five to six years ago, a couple or so years after Kennan had left medical practice. As I was collating the material, he asked for a pause, because he felt there may be too much reactionary comment to the material. When I asked him why, he gave the expected answer of his recent departure from practice, but then informed me that his marriage and various business interests needed attention, and the work may have been, and could become, coloured by this process.

Reluctantly, I agreed to the pause, believing it would only be a matter of months. But then it lengthened. I moved to other projects and Kennan showed no interest in completing the project. Then in a two-year period, he had divested himself of his business interests and his marriage had dissolved. He also explained that he had a stint in hospital with a heart complaint when Covid first surfaced and that this experience, as well as the ensuing drama of the pandemic, had galvanised him. He ridded himself of any superfluous assets and moved to a retreat den in a forest region; there he appeared to have retired from any professional interest beyond his spiritual activities and some counselling work.

We had kept up personal contact, but I had presumed this work was in indefinite mothballs. Then I received a call when the Covid pandemic started to wane from its initial onslaught. Kennan surprised me as he suggested we edit the existing mothballed material and get to publication. He told me that we could add more insights derived from this intervening period beyond practice, with his further experience and reflections. He felt he wanted to "get the story out there".

I willingly agreed. And, at the same time, any lingering doubts I had about the man's motives, intentions and integrity also finally and completely dissipated.

One

I felt a long way from home. The young woman's pulse was strong and regular. The owner of the pulse was only eighteen, of ethnic origin, and in a coma induced by an overdose of drugs. Her long black hair framed an obviously Mediterranean face from which calm, peace and beauty seemed to radiate almost in spite of herself, or so it seemed to me at the time. She was breathing regularly in spite of all the activity in the large ward and the array of equipment around her, and her pulse was regular and strong.

I was a resident medical doctor in a major teaching hospital in Perth, Western Australia and I was really pissed off. It was Friday night and I was on rostered call for the night, as I was every Friday when the other doctors downed stethoscopes and gathered for an in-house so-called Happy Hour. Instead, I was making the rounds of patients who needed a last check – tucking in – before going to the doctor's lounge for some tea and television, so avoiding the smell of beer emanating from the refectory.

"You won't let her die, will you doctor?" came a voice from a chair in the corner, some distance from the bed. I had not noticed anyone else in the immediate vicinity of the bed when I first entered. And in that very moment she did die. I felt her pulse suddenly cease and I looked up at her face. She was no longer breathing. The resuscitation team was there in less than a minute, but to no avail. The tearlessly sobbing mother gave me one last scathing look as she left the ward. The look confused and hurt me at the time, but then I inwardly reacted: "You fucking bitch, you killed her!" ... to myself, of course.

At the time, I was shocked to the core by this event. I knew that the patient had somehow heard her mother's voice and decided to leave, to die. I knew this in her pulse as it stopped. And I knew from the accusatory demand of the mother's question that this young woman had had enough. She was going home; although I only fully realised all of this many years later.

I felt a yawning gap beneath me; a void had opened up. What had happened then and there? Maybe now, with the maturity of years, I can answer that question. But at this early stage in my career, I just felt the certainty and security of the profession I had chosen ripped away from underneath me. She had died. We couldn't prevent that with all our knowledge and equipment. Something bigger had happened, something bigger than all my training.

I eventually came to the conclusion that the patient realised her mother was there, and that her mother was somehow the reason for the overdose. She wanted to escape, maybe not to die, but just to get away from her mother or the family. I didn't know her story; she was not my patient. Had she tried before and failed? Was there a boyfriend who had deserted her? Where was the father? Why was she taking drugs? Was she an addict?

There were no immediately ready-made answers to these questions. The circumstantial ones worried me at the time, but the larger ones crept in over the ensuing years. How did she 'know' her mother was there? She was in a coma; did she 'hear' her? And, if so, how? How could she 'decide' to die? All I felt was that she was going somewhere more peaceful. I call it home.

And then I realised, in that moment, that I was also a long way from home. But where and what is that home?

Kennan and I met periodically to discuss his life and work. I am a writer, author and university lecturer. I had strong leanings toward health and its delivery born of my own chronic illness and subsequent dealings with the medical establishment. I had only come to know him as a client in his writing ventures in the latter part of his medical career, when his vision already seemed beyond formal medical practice. It was not until he left practice that this changed to a more earnest desire on his part for us to work together on a memoir, rather than the joint project we had planned when we first met.

I realised, even then, that I was being used. The memoir was a ruse to deal creatively with leaving a profession he had once held dear; he wanted a trade as a wordsmith now. But was he manipulating me? Was he a psychopath? I didn't know the answers then, but I was willing to go along for the ride, for the time being, at least. If my fingers started to get burned, I could always leave, I reasoned.

So, we started.

The meetings were in varied locations, usually cafés where I could have a notepad and tape voice recordings, if needed, as well as ask questions to fill in any details or gaps in his account, as I perceived them.

I was somewhat surprised about the story he used to start this account. I had expected a chronological narrative, but Kennan explained that this story kept beckoning after years in the wilderness of his memory, so he followed his intuition and started there. This was an initial and ongoing feature; that he would move around his journey in a seemingly haphazard way, and I would sometimes be floundering trying to fill in gaps. He would reassure me about this approach, maintaining that we would – inevitably – cover what was necessary. His implicit trust in this more intuitive approach was already a distinguishing feature.

As were the more prophetic aspects of his account. It seemed, on many occasions, that he anticipated changes that were to occur in medical thinking and its direction. At first, I questioned whether this was just the benefit of hindsight, but the integrity of the accounts at the time made me realise this was probably not the case. It seemed Kennan had a genuine ability in being able to predict what would "come to pass", so to speak. As will be seen, this would be put to the test toward the end of this account, when I challenged him on some predictions of medicine's future.

It also made me realise how much at odds Kennan was and would become to his colleagues, as well as the profession at large. This kind of perception and resulting worldview can be viewed with awe in the knowledge of significant figures from history, but, at the time, it is a difficult position to maintain in the face of orthodoxy. Although not to the same degree as Kennan, I had experienced something similar at various times in my own teaching career. It was not surprising that we should have large areas of compatibility, otherwise why would I now be interviewing him? And why would he otherwise trust me with his story? Maybe he wasn't a psychopath after all, I concluded. But this was not the first time my feelings would oscillate in such a dramatic manner.

I had asked Kennan early on why he was not relating this account directly; why had he chosen me to do it? The flattery about my writing skills and teaching abilities was appreciated, but I was not seduced with the explanation; I felt there were other reasons. Maybe he believed that his story would not be appreciated were he to relate it directly. Or maybe he felt it added a level of obfuscation that protected the content. I remained unsure as to which, if either, or even other reasons at this early stage in our adventure.

I also asked him about the significance of his personal life in the account, as he related little about relationships and family. His response was interesting, although a little predictable: He felt that he should only include his personal life, and that of his family, if it was directly relevant to the account itself from a health and medical perspective. This firm boundary seemed to dissipate as we progressed, as it proved impossible to dismiss the influence of his personal journey on his professional life; in fact, it was and is an essential component. As will become apparent, this personal story is not insignificant, as it involves serious illnesses he experienced, as well as the death of the mother to two of his children. It also included his relationship and difficulties with alcohol.

Kennan also wondered that too much personal input would detract from the narrative and allow for criticisms that would obscure what he was trying to convey – as if he knew clearly what that was! However, I was more discerning in that respect, and he had given me license. Yet this divide became apparent when we were to discuss sexuality in relation to health and medicine. Whilst Kennan's own relatively wide and varied sexual experience gave him insights and a deeper understanding of the role of sex in health and medicine, it could be an easy subject for commentators to analyse and criticise with respect to his personal disposition and motives. Therefore, I decided to let this personal censoring issue drop and see how things emerged, as I reasoned that Kennan's position may change as we progressed

– changeability is in the very nature of the man, I concluded.

There was a paradox here. I was to discover that in his therapeutic and educational approaches, such as workshops and retreats, he would often open up significantly about his personal life. Somehow these settings facilitated such revelation, because they were not viewed in the same critical and judgmental manner, but as metaphors and symbols of wisdom. Maybe not a psychopath, but a narcissist? Bugger me, was I already charmed! Back to the account…

> It wasn't entirely as a result of the preceding event that my career changed but, with the wisdom of years, I can now see how my faith in modern medicine was permanently undermined in that moment. I can also see that there were warning signs of this throughout my training with other such moments, and I would have cause to reflect on these as my career progressed. But there I was, right at the beginning of that career, having qualified some months before, and undertaking my hospital residency. I had set sail, so changing direction this early on was not something I had entertained or even thought about.
>
> Some factual information: Medical qualifications with the passing of examinations does not allow a fledgling doctor to direct practice with the public straightaway. To do this, he or she must undertake a period of supervised practice in an accredited institution. In my case, this was in Perth, Western Australia, as a pre-registration resident doctor. This supervised period is for a minimum of one year, after the satisfactory completion of which the doctor becomes a registered medical practitioner. He or she is then free to practice without the constraints of the pre-registration period, although this perceived autonomy

is now relative and becoming less so, to the point of extinction. In fact, with the development of general practice as a specialty and demanding further training, it is almost impossible.

At the time of the above event, I was at the beginning of my registration year in Australia, although my upbringing and training had been in England. My family had emigrated whilst I was studying at Oxford University, although, as a family, we had spent two years living in Perth prior to this, during my teenage years. Later in my training in England, the career opportunities appeared better in Australia, so after I qualified, I undertook my registration here, which would also allow me to practice in either country. However, because of my prior teenage experience here, I already saw the move as permanent, and my fledgling family had also agreed to settle in Australia.

I was now a resident on the psychiatric ward for a portion of this required pre-registration period, although, at this stage of my career, psychiatry was not at all to my liking. I had just completed a stint in the casualty section of the hospital, where I had enjoyed the action and practicality of applying my trade. In contrast, psychiatry seemed dull, and I could not see its relevance to either medicine or my future. I saw it as unnecessary, an intrusion onto my projected career path. However, it put me in a frame of mind to question the woman's death more than I might otherwise.

Somehow during that registration year, when the years of training were put into supervised practice, the fledgling graduate was meant to decide a career future, if it had not already been determined during the training years, or by other more social factors. I had always gravitated to the practical side of medicine. A farmer's son, I am used to seeing the results of my endeavours and it seemed then that a career in surgery would fulfil these expectations.

But the young woman's death haunted me with deeper questions about health that surfaced, as I started the selection process for specialist surgical training. Then I had an insight: I decided to meet in person the three surgical teaching professors in the hospital system and ask them about my career choice. Overtly, this was to see if my application would be treated favourably, as well as to display my enthusiasm; but the covert reason was to explore what the future outcome of such a career choice might look like for me.

I was dismayed by these meetings, though strangely not completely surprised – it was almost as if I had expected this outcome. One was an academic boffin; the other two were clinically depressed, in my opinion – I was doing psychiatry at the time, after all. All would support my application, but did I want to end up like them at their stage of career? My misgivings led to a choice: I withdrew my application.

Where would I turn then? I had become registered by this stage so could go into private practice – not a choice now at this point in a medical career – so I decided to continue with residency positions at the hospital; effectively, I was treading water. The positions I was subsequently given were not of my request and, I surmised, these were a reaction from the hospital administration for my wanting to pursue specialist training, rather than continuing with rotating post-registration residency positions. Even though I had been open and explained my intentions to the administrative doctor making such allocations, they had obviously been inconvenienced, or I was caught in some unknown internal politics and this was payback. This struck me as unethical, but what could I do? I swallowed my pride and took the next rostered position in a regional hospital in Kalgoorlie, mainly because I had a sense of adventure about this posting in the perceived Wild West of Western Australia.

It was possibly a surprise that Kennan had come this far in his medical career, as in some ways he seemed to be ill-suited to the profession and not focused in either what he wanted or expected from it. His background was entirely non-medical, although health had always intrigued him. But it was the difference between health itself and its expression in modern medicine that was to trouble him throughout his career, endorsed by his innate spiritual inclinations.

Somewhat naïvely, Kennan considered medicine to be an extension of health where illness and disease were to be rectified, when necessary, and a balance of health re-established and fostered. This is what he had experienced on the farm as a boy, where health preservation was the main focus. The role of the veterinarian was to maintain the overall health in the livestock. Illness was seen as necessitating treatment and support to restore health, and if disease were not remedial then an animal was allowed to die, or put down if suffering. This appreciation was further endorsed and reinforced at Oxford University in attaining his physiology degrees with academic teachers.

On the farm, much attention was placed on good husbandry. The welfare of the animals was founded on such fundamentals as good food and a healthy environment. Support was given in times of need, such as additional feed and shelter in winter.

Animals were tended to – nursed – when unwell and the Vet only brought in if health was not naturally restored in a reasonable period of time. In a farm with many kinds of animals, the community was important and there were specific roles. The cats kept the vermin down and the dogs retrieved any rabbits or game shot, or were bred for profit.

As children, Kennan and his siblings flowed into and were part of this community. Many animals, and not just the cats and dogs, had names and identifiable personalities. The children grieved if one died, were happy when they bred, and laughed at their sexual antics. Birth, sex, and death were an integral part of the farm and community, and Kennan was involved in all of them from an early age. Death, most particularly, was something he was exposed to and did not fear at this relative arm's length.

Kennan had a wide-ranging native intelligence and did well at school. This opened up avenues of academia and intellectual inquiry that were in many ways incompatible with farm life as a future career. As the only son, he was in a position to inherit the farm and its lifestyle, but early on he chose not to. For all its health and vitality, it was a hard life and his schooling to date indicated more attractive choices beyond the farm.

> I was asked early on: Why did I choose medicine? I will explain a little here; although Ian might have been able to do this better than I, he did allow me my unedited voice at this point, if well-reasoned. Big of him.
>
> Maybe it was a naïve choice, but it didn't seem so at the time – it felt inspired. Although I had already gained a place at Oxford University, I was unsure about a career beyond a degree. The choice of medicine was made in a sudden moment of clarity after talking to some colleagues, when I realised that medicine may

satisfy my intellectual and community interests, as well as having practical application. Little did I know that medicine may satisfy the latter, but ultimately not the former two aspects. I could have done with some mentoring at that time; maybe my father was angry with my decision not to follow him, and instead he had produced two further daughters. Karma?

I did not realise all this in my three years at Oxford, where the college system meant that medical students mixed with students of all other disciplines. In my academic year, the college had three medical students, myself included, within a student body of over one hundred. My intellectual and social exposure was wide and varied. It was also not primarily medical; the three years at Oxford were in the wider context of a degree in physiological sciences whilst also satisfying the so-called pre-clinical medical requirements, prior to going into the clinical hospital setting to complete training.

Doctors do a minimum requirement of physiology in their training. This is a great shame, in my opinion. What physiology provides is a much broader perspective of the body beyond illness and disease. In fact, it is not focused on illness; physiology is primarily concerned with the normal functioning of the body, or organism, and hence with wellbeing in the broadest sense. Exposure to physiology in more detail can also develop a respect in the student for the body's normal functioning, its self-regulation, and capacity to naturally deal with imbalance, including illness and even its place in disease states.

These principles accorded well with my experiences on the family farm. So, I could enjoy the rich and varied life that Oxford provided with plenty of sex, alcohol and rock n' roll, without having any qualms about medicine as my career choice. I flirted with other disciplines, like psychology and philosophy, and was tempted to do a doctorate in neurophysiology after I completed my primary degree. The life at Oxford appealed, but I was now engaged to be married and it seemed time to get a job.

Everything came to a grinding emotional halt when I started my clinical studies at St Bartholomew's Hospital in London. Thrust onto large wards full of sick people was a culture shock and then, for the first time, I seriously doubted my career choice. I became desperate and a bit lost, so I phoned our local family general practitioner where I had grown up. He had since become a mentor of sorts, and on his advice, I took leave to spend some time with him to try and find my feet and direction.

Brian was the general practitioner of a group of villages in the English Midlands, which included the farm I was brought up on. I now gained a view of medicine in general practice life that was rich, varied, and rewarding. This was, and is, the kind of medicine I found attractive. I still do.

I did house calls with Brian. He knew the communities and was socially embedded in them. He knew patients by their Christian names, had delivered and helped raise their families, and many were friends. He had seen them through hardship and helped bury their dead. He was respected and valued by the community. There was then little political interference and certainly little sense of medicolegal medicine, except around such matters as sexuality.

I sat with Brian through his consultations. Had Brian informed anyone in authority that this was happening? I doubt it. He sometimes got me to start a surgery. This, mind you, was after a mere two months on the wards of clinical medicine. But I found I could cope. My confidence grew, I could see a place for myself, and I decided I liked medicine again.

There are many stories, such as the old lady who came in with a lump on her head. Brian gently squeezed it and expressed the paste that is contained within a sebaceous cyst. The lump disappeared.

"Thank you doctor!" she said, with a tear in her eye.

"Brian," I said, after she had departed and being the smartass, "you know that will come back sooner or later?"

"Yes," he said, "and then I'll do it again!"

Although I couldn't put my finger on exactly what at the time, I knew I had learned something important.

There was the complaining man with his shopping list of symptoms. Brian patiently listened and scribbled 'NTFA' on his notepad so that I could see it. When – eventually – the consultation ended, I asked Brian what NTFA meant, because I had been racking my brains for a medical illness that fitted the acronym.

Brian simply replied, with a smile on his face "A nasty touch of fuck all!"

I squirmed a little, but not as much as when Brian repeated the scribbling with a little old lady of a similar disposition an hour or so later. I felt like a schoolboy giggling in class and having to hide it!

What I was most grateful for is witnessing my first birth. Brian had engineered this event so that it would be a home birth at a local farmhouse. It was Mum's fourth, so little intervention was necessary. Dad fed the other kids downstairs.

"It'll be a girl," he said, "usually is when the cows

are overdue".

He was right. And I wept that deep guttural weeping that is so moving and life-changing. It was and still is one of the most beautiful experiences of my life. After a few weeks, I returned to London, determined now to finish my training and become a doctor – like Brian, of course.

Bugger me! Now that I write and reflect on this, I wonder whether Brian had done me a disservice. Maybe he was expecting me to live out his unfulfilled ambition? I think there's an element of that. I reckon now he would say: "Get the hell out of it!"

It was at this point in our discussion that Kennan felt that he wanted to reflect on some of the issues that had come up in the narrative to date. For example, he thought that the experience of being raised on an English farm was more important than he had realised. The nature of the farm itself, being mixed with grain farming and various animals – chickens, pigs, sheep, cows, even exotic rabbits – provided an important basis for health of a more communal, social and environmental nature. In other words, it was holistic, as was any veterinarian healthcare involvement.

This was reflected in Brian's medical practice which encompassed a group of rural villages, so that it provided a familiar background for Kennan. However, at this stage in his narrative, Kennan began to realise the lack of input and direction he had received from others in his career choices. Instead, he had relied on his innate intelligence that often lacked the depth of experience necessary for wisdom in such choices. In hindsight, he believes he would have left any medical career after finishing his degree at Oxford and continued in academic and research life but, as well as the prospect of an impending marriage and its attendant responsibilities, Brian's influence had been pivotal.

As were Kennan's experiences in London. While we talked, we wondered whether every generation would feel the acute sense of transition that Kennan had felt in the profession over his time in it. In summary, he sees this change to be from an art to a science. This is a topic we returned to in our discussions, sometimes frequently, although it did seem to us that we had witnessed a significant and accelerated change that has not yet abated. This leaves us both with a concerned outlook for the place of modern medicine in future healthcare. I know Kennan believes that medicine has gone past a critical point, and that the necessary changes that healthcare needs to go through will not be spearheaded by modern medicine itself.

At this stage of his career, such speculation was obviously not part of his worldview; it was premature. What Brian had instilled in Kennan was a focus that, to achieve what he wanted, he would have to embrace modern medicine in its fullest, and then leave it to later times to make choices in and any modifications to this. We shall see as the story unfolds that these would be varied and plentiful, but ultimately led to an incompatibility with the medical profession as it exists in the modern era.

Kennan also reflected on two areas that were to vex and trouble him at various points throughout his career. The first was sexuality. It is not that there appeared to be anything untoward about Kennan's sexuality, it is just that he has found it difficult to reconcile sexuality within his profession. In general, he sees that sexuality is a hidden and dismissed undercurrent in medicine at both personal and professional levels. This is ironic, as it has a considerable part to play in health, illness, and even disease.

Interests of this sort, and Kennan's progressive recognition of their undercurrents in practice, were one of the main reasons his orientation moved to the more psychological and psychiatric areas of medicine as his experience in practice increased. It was here, of course, that he found Freud, and many others who were also following this line of inquiry, not only in history but also the present. The problem as he saw it, and still sees it, is that sexuality has now all but been eliminated from medical discussion and certainly the one that exists between doctor and patient.

This is a huge topic, one that I have expressed in various writings over the years. Yet this is more than purely academic; it is a practical and fundamental feature of health and wellbeing. And it is lacking in the medical mainstream. Kennan's opinion is that, for this reason alone, modern medicine lacks the seeds of renewal of healthcare that the future will demand. Why? Because in Kennan's words, "sex is fundamentally all about renewal."

Beyond a certain point this could become such a major theme of this narrative that I believe Kennan and I needed to be careful. Certainly, there will be stories about sex and medicine in what is to follow. But the wider implications of this, such as an examination of sex in disease or the sexuality that exists between patient and practitioner, would take us too far afield at this time. Yet as we discussed this – and the discussions were frank and wide-ranging – we decided it might become a future work and, if not, it should.

The second area was alcohol. Not only has Kennan had a longstanding relationship with alcohol, but also, like all relationships, this has undergone changes throughout his lifetime. Alcohol usage preceded medical practice for Kennan. It was an integral part of his social life and one he was brought up in. With Brian's input, he received not only an education in medicine as an art, but also an appreciation of fine wines.

Ultimately the use or misuse of alcohol was a factor in his

decision to leave medical practice. This theme, along with other associated areas, will weave its way through this work in a significant manner. Ironically, one thing that will become apparent is that one reason modern medicine is not well is because its practitioners are not well; they are often medicating themselves to an alarming degree, and not just with alcohol.

Two

Kennan had been unwell following our initial meetings. After a brief overseas holiday to Bali, he had returned with the flu, which progressed to a chest infection and subsequently a viral pneumonia. At least that was his assessment. If I put a medical hat on, it sounded remarkably like SARS to me. And now, more than five years later and as I put the finishing touches to this work, it seems to have anticipated the Covid pandemic crisis that has recently gripped – Kennan would say 'entranced' – the world.

True to his beliefs, Kennan insisted that there was no clinical indication for it being more than a viral infection. He didn't want unnecessary tests, and was also in contact with an old medical colleague, James, so he decided to continue with symptomatic measures with this support in the wings. When I made a comment about whether he had considered using an antibiotic, I received a chilling stare and no reply. I decided not to persist.

As the illness lingered on, I felt nervous. Kennan explained to me that he often experienced complications with common upper respiratory afflictions like a common cold, and that he invariably developed chest problems. Usually this was a troublesome bronchitis, but on this occasion, it was both more severe, painful and persistent. He felt that was because he had contracted it abroad and that it had followed a period of undue personal stress.

Kennan then explained to me that, as a child, he was considered to have a hearing problem. Indeed, his first conscious memory was of being in a hospital bed after he had had his tonsils and adenoids removed. The justification for this operation had been that 'catarrh' build-up was contributing to his deafness and that removing these seemingly unnecessary organs would help his hearing. The justification was invalid. It made no difference. Kennan was then to have other interventions, such as repeated clearing of his upper hearing passages and even irradiation of his sinuses. In hindsight, this all seems medieval, even barbaric. But his parents acquiesced; they were young, and the authority of the doctor was sacrosanct.

Kennan's later interpretation was that he was deaf because he didn't want to listen to the difficulties this young couple, his parents, were going through. This failure to listen was probably more psychic than physical, in his opinion. I wondered how autistic he might be assessed to have been today. I know it has also caused him to follow the current argument about autism, so-called spectrum disorders, and vaccination usage with more than a passing interest. As a child, he recalls a very strong and irrational resistance to any vaccination beyond any discomfort that it may have caused him.

Were autism to have been the case, then he would now probably receive much more in the way of psychological and social therapy. Yet, at that time, physical intervention was predominant, as it was in many overlapping physical and psychological areas such as this. It was a time, on a wave of scientific success, when medicine had a primarily mechanical outlook that is only now slowly changing, although still with an ambivalence and more than a little confusion with its direction in these intersecting positions.

Although Kennan had been left with the legacy of all this, he decided not to compound the problem with further medical management that may be found not to be in his best health interests. Rather, he accepted what had happened and now manages the consequences as naturally and supportively as he is able. He remains acutely aware of his respiratory system in his overall physical and psychological makeup. Interestingly, he believes that many of the lingering problems in this area have largely resolved since then; confirmed by him with a query from me, some years after that specific chest illness.

In Kennan's opinion, this illness was somehow a necessity. He did elaborate on some of the personal stressors that contributed to it, but at this stage in our inquiry he asked me not to reveal them, so remaining true to his original injunction about differentiating the personal and professional issues in this account. I found the issue of 'necessity' difficult to follow at the time, as might the reader at this point in the narrative; but over time I gained a better appreciation, as I understood his spiritual position from a more shamanic perspective. When this realisation occurred for me, I also found that the apparent separation of the personal from the professional seemed to diminish; I guess he then trusted me more.

We went on to discuss the issue of the change in modern medicine's position over his years in practice and beyond in some detail, because it seemed significant to us that there had been a rapid and sometimes dramatic change in emphasis. Medicine, like many disciplines, evolves, but is also governed by factors outside of its immediate influence. The fact that, when Kennan was a child, the world was seen in a more mechanical manner was reflected in the medical view of illness at that time. This has now become more technological, although in both our views, this is really more of the same. A more psychosocial outlook is emerging, which we both deem significant, and this will be an important consideration when we come to look at the future of health and medicine; not simply within medicine, but also its integration with the broader and more psychospiritual domain of health, healing and wellbeing.

The next story that Kennan told exemplified this issue. Yet it also pointed to something even greater: The role and disposition of the individual in health and wellbeing. Although embryonic in this story, this issue was not to become a conscious feature for many years, until Kennan moved into psychological areas of medicine.

> Over time, I became accepting of my place in hospital training and the demands that would fulfil my ambition of qualifying as a doctor. I also accepted, at this time, the rigours of digesting the mountain of information necessary to get through the incessant checks and examinations. But I soon realised I had an inevitably inquiring mind that is open to the unusual, the facts that don't fit, and stories that portend more than the obvious.
>
> St Bartholomew's Hospital – or Barts – was, and is, a venerable institution. Certainly, one of the world's oldest hospital and teaching institutions, it was replete with tradition, which I still find appealing and important. The staff there included consultant specialists who spent most of their time in the renowned Harley Street, when not teaching. They told stories, lots of stories. And these stories were to inexplicably then satisfy me whilst I simultaneously absorbed, digested, and regurgitated the facts and information fed to the students by the younger training specialists.
>
> I was one of about eight students seated in a row some ten feet from the large desk that faced us, and behind which was seated the specialist obstetrician. He was Canadian and the author in a standard textbook on the subject for we medical students. Likeable and good humoured, he would bring in a pregnant woman

and seat her, facing us and to his right, before discussing her condition.

On this occasion, he brought in a more mature woman of commanding appearance and with an associated air of confidence. He explained to us that, although in her thirties, this was her first pregnancy and she was having twins. He asked us to consider how we would manage the case, and his gaze settled on a colleague to my left:

"I would consider a Caesarean section, sir."

"And why would you consider this?"

"Because of the age of the mother; being her first pregnancy, and the potential complications, sir."

"You don't think she can give birth vaginally then? And I haven't even got to breast-feeding," he said with a suppressed chuckle.

My colleague, oblivious to the potential import of the chuckle, then went into a detailed explanation of the risks associated with a vaginal delivery, repeating his concerns about her age and first pregnancy. All this time the mother-to-be sat unmoved and with a quiet smile.

The consultant intervened: "I think there is something you ought to know. This young woman rowed single-handedly across the Atlantic. I think she will be more than capable of delivering and breast feeding her children normally." He then escorted the rower behind a curtain, where he examined her and, with his customary charm, showed her to the door. She had said not a word nor adjusted her demeanour through the whole encounter barring the odd smile. She then thanked him directly on her departure with a look of admiration.

This simple statement provided the kind of

information that I found so interesting. It encapsulated my awareness of the two sides of medicine. On the one hand being the science and associated skills, technology, and information that modern medicine could bring to any given situation. But on the other, it also pointed to the dimensions beyond, such as the psychological and social, and how important it was to consider these in the equation and any medical management.

Kennan had picked a story well into his clinical training. I was sure there were others that preceded it. He assured me there were and that we might well return to some, but he recalled this particular story at this time because of a further point it illustrated.

Within the disposition and demeanour of the woman existed qualities Kennan could only guess at and infer. And these qualities had an impact on her condition – if pregnancy could be reasonably considered a medical condition – and its management. It would be easy to ignore these generally, although maybe not so with this particular woman! And it is often the case that medicine does ignore them; yet the attitudes, beliefs and values of a person, or patient, have or should have a significant bearing on any decision regarding management.

Ultimately this comes down to something relatively intangible, and that is the personality, temperament, or some inherent quality of the patient. This has somehow to be accommodated and assessed, but how to do this? And can it be done objectively, or does it require the skill or art of the practitioner, partially or maybe entirely? This question was to remain with Kennan, and it would be nearly a decade before it emerged with more force and significance, and mainly because of what he was going through in his personal life.

There are other dimensions to this story. It harkened back to his days at Oxford where physiology had taught Kennan about the body's inherent wisdom. And further that we were still discovering, understanding and appreciating this wisdom, so to supersede it with our scientific knowledge that was limited in both content and scope illustrated an arrogance that humans are guilty of, and all too frequently.

With the pregnant woman, it was easy. She could go into labour and then we have the tools of medicine available, should things go awry. But we should not presume they would. Nor should we necessarily interfere because they might. There was a deeper level to this inquiry that slowly dawned on Kennan, and it was more spiritual in nature. This woman was blessed with twins and maybe it was because she could have them, and her body knew this. Also, irrespective of the outcome, this was her lot, her choice. This all started to get a little deep and hazy for Kennan, so he parked this line of thinking, although it would return.

Kennan was drawn to the divide between physiology and pathology. Where was the dividing line? And was it up to us, as doctors, to assess and decide it? Couldn't it be both, as in his outline of allowing nature first and then medicine if we get into difficulty? Isn't that what traditional approaches do? Kennan cast his mind around his experiences to date and settled on two stories that maybe took this inquiry further.

> Earlier in my training I recall standing next to a bed in the large ward occupied by an appropriately large man. I was one of about a dozen students with our teaching consultant, who were also gathered around the bed. Prior to this particular event, each student would have been nominated a patient in the ward and conducted an interview with him or her, in the manner

of a trainee doctor. This consisted of asking about the story of the malaise – the history – and then a physical examination. At times one of we students was then called upon to present this to the consultant, usually in front of our peers, as was occurring here.

I recall on this occasion that it was a male student who was recounting the history, which all my colleagues were listening to intently, because of the inevitable questions that would follow from the consultant to others around the bed. My colleague presented the case, and I cannot now recall what was wrong with the man. But I do recall that, when the history came to the section entitled 'social history', my colleague said:

"Mr Jones is an alcoholic." He made this statement seemingly oblivious to the man in the bed. However, the large man turned not a hair.

"On what do you base this assessment?" asked the consultant.

"Well, sir, he often drinks over twelve pints of beer a day. And many of these are at lunchtime."

"This man works ... where?"

"On the docks, sir."

A long pause: "Well, let me tell you that it is quite normal for a docker to drink twelve or more pints of beer a day, if he is so inclined. This man is not an alcoholic."

The patient smiled, but I was confused. I recalled the lecture about alcohol and alcoholism. In this I was given the impression that alcoholism had two dimensions. The first was dependence, which was given a more physical basis around craving and the like. This patient seemed not to display this, as his transition into hospital to have his complaint dealt with was not accompanied by any withdrawal symptoms. The second was abuse, which was more psychological. In a direct manner, the consultant was pointing out that the context of his drinking was not abusive, that it was somehow normal. This was obviously more complex and open to question, although I was inclined to accept the consultant's judgement, based on his experience. Maybe this reflects my own preferences, however?

So, was the lecture wrong? Probably not, although I noticed over the years that alcohol and alcoholism is a constantly changing picture, and not always based on clear and cold medical facts. It was and is that the social, environmental, and cultural factors had an impact that were often minimised, sometimes ignored in medicine generally. After all, areas like 'social history' were right at the end of the history-taking procedure and most frequently the documented entry was 'nil relevant'. I confess to personal interest both past and present here.

This story had features that did not impact directly on the condition the patient had. It wasn't alcohol-related; hence the disparity of labelling the man with a second disease – alcoholism – to add to his medical history was inappropriate in the consultant's eyes, when it was an inherent part of his social pattern and those around him. Maybe it would be considered 'appropriate' now though? Maybe also, it is too early to go down that rabbit hole …

However, I found it an interesting story for Kennan to choose in response to a query about the relationship between physiology and pathology. It seemed more about the relationship between pathology and social habits, rather than physiological disturbance. I wondered more about the current significance for Kennan and whether that had affected his choice of story. I was tempted to edit this story out of the account, when I had a second thought; maybe Kennan is revealing something of himself with this story, so I decided to include it and stay tuned in. I was moving away from trying to diagnose this man with a personality disorder, I reflected.

Something else I had decided to do was not to remove Kennan's account of factual issues in training and practice. Of course, with my detailed interest in healthcare I could do this, keeping his account to the stories and other spicier elements. This would help to contrast our styles and build up some tension, mainly for the reader. But I decided not to use this ploy, because it felt mildly deceitful. In ways we are very alike, so the subtlety of any differences would be present and make the account more authentic, in my opinion. The consequence of this would be that the two accounts would sometimes seem to overlap, even merge. Then again, maybe I have allowed him to seduce me with his verbal charm …

> The aspiring doctors' next consultant had a permanently stiff leg. He had been shot in the knee during the war. A tall lean man, he still walked in a commanding way as he entered the small room in which we students were gathered. He sat at the head and swung his stiff leg onto the table: "I remember a story!"
>
> This was how he commonly started, as he often eschewed the so-called ward round and favoured the repartee in gatherings such as this. At the time, the students often found this inconvenient, because they wanted information for the inevitably looming next examination stage of their training, whilst I was of a mixed opinion. Instead, we had this Harley Street icon

telling us stories. Yet, I reflected, I now recall none of the facts dispensed by the feverish trainee specialists in the same room on the expansive blackboard. But I do recall many or most of the stories.

The story was of a teenage girl at school who started to get fat. Well, it wasn't obesity; it was a distinct swelling of her lower belly, or abdomen. She was the daughter of the Minister of Sport and attended a prestigious girls' school, and the problem was that the staff and then doctors declared the obesity to be the consequence of pregnancy, unbeknownst to her. Shock, horror, embarrassment! But what to do? Disguise it as long as possible, so it doesn't become public. Our patient is well, but when she continues to swell yet play immaculate hockey passed her due by date, it is decided she has must have a tumour and be investigated; hence her presence in the ward.

I am aware that this particular situation would never have come to this point in the present medical era, yet sometimes the obvious is bypassed for a plethora of other reasons, so it is more a metaphor. For example, I recall, and will shortly return to, a story of seeing a young woman in a casualty ward referred by her family's local general practitioner with suspected appendicitis. When I came to examine her, I discovered that the source of her pain was that she was in the early stages of labour.

So, the bright young heroine of this current story is in bed with her tumour when the consultant arrives. This man was an alcoholic, so visits were rare and usually just a routine, even a courtesy and acknowledgement of maybe his prior status and contribution to the profession. He was then escorted around the ward after a social chat in the nurses' station. And it was escorting, because the specialists and trainees underneath him in the pecking order were fully aware of the situation and simply supported it, because he was near retirement and so they managed the ward themselves.

"Unfortunate case this, sir," was how his second-in-command started, "probable terminal ovarian cancer admitted for diagnosis and further investigation."

"You fools!" was the consultant's response, "don't you recognise an ovarian cyst when you see one?" Although I doubt this statement was delivered with the venom that was relayed to us! The next day she was delivered of a ten-kilogram plus ovarian cyst.

Kennan had begun this story intending to illustrate further the blurred boundary between pathology and physiology. Although, technically the cyst is not physiological, it is actually an extension of normal physiology; it occurs when something goes amiss with the normal hormonal control of the cyclic process and a cyst results. Sometimes, as in this situation, they can be massive.

The message from the consultant was about this distinction and the assumptions that had been made, but there was also more. It illustrated a principle in medicine about the so-called special patient, how they can be managed differently, and the problems that can result from this. In this respect the problem is obvious, but maybe Kennan recalled this story because of the 'special' way his pregnant partner was dealt with many years later, with disastrous consequences.

As he reflected on this tale now, Kennan is amused about the alcohol component of the story. He recalls that this was recounted with no judgement about the alcoholic consultant; what seemed to be emphasised in an indirect kind of manner was that the man's experience was still recognised and valid. I also wondered whether it was some kind of mythic metaphor about his own recent experiences and the manner with which they were dealt. There was a large part of the confessional embedded in Kennan's account, particularly the stories. In what way might this be distorting the memoir, I pondered? But rather than bring this point up I decided to just let it be and see where his further account took us in this meandering journey.

The young girl with the 'appendicitis' though! Kennan laughed. At the time he was surprised, but not astounded. That the girl did not know – she was fifteen and from a rural village and working-family's household – was not altogether a surprise. But neither did her mother, who was also present. Maybe she was in denial, thought Kennan. Anyway, he was a surgical resident and not an obstetrician, so a phone call to a colleague was in order.

But what about the general practitioner? Kennan surmised that he had not seen the patient and had just made a presumptive diagnosis to get her to casualty. Was he avoiding a house call? May he be otherwise occupied, so unable to attend? Kennan was never to know. Yet this obfuscation in medicine around matters sexual was an interest that was aroused in the latter part of his training, when students were finally exposed to the gynaecology wards.

> I recall the woman in the hospital bed being investigated for primary infertility after two years of marriage. It often requires that sort of time period before medicine is engaged in situations like this, which is extremely sad when the outcome of this particular story is revealed.
>
> Here she was occupying the bed of a London Teaching Hospital for investigation. Our consultant

was a meticulous man. He wore a bow tie and spent several minutes talking to the patient about the magazine she'd been reading while in bed. As we shuffled our feet he then, somewhat surprisingly, abruptly terminated the interview without engaging an expected medical inquiry and we moved elsewhere.

Here, in a private area, he informed us that the reason that she had not fallen pregnant was because both she and her husband believed pregnancy occurred when the man's semen is deposited in the woman's navel. So, they had been trying for a pregnancy in this manner for two years and were distraught that she had not conceived.

Two years! And a simple yet thorough inquiry would have obviated the delay and the psychological distress. Yet nobody had conducted this inquiry. It was the consultant's job to deal with this as a result. He wasn't going to kick her out of the expensive bed with a couple of pamphlets or shirk his responsibility. The chat about the magazine was part of what would unfold. As she responded to his overtures and had developed what medicine calls a rapport, he would take the time to go back and counsel her and her husband. To me, this is the art of medicine in action.

Yet the consultant had another side (don't we all?). He could be quite blunt and frank. At a later ward round, he and the students spent time with a woman who was being investigated for pelvic pain. With the husband present, he managed to skillfully and without embarrassment elicit much about her sex life, personal attitudes and beliefs. It was a consummate performance.

Then he gathered we students into a quiet area: "What do you think is wrong with this patient, gentlemen?" And we were just male students on this occasion, probably appropriately with what was to follow. Initially, we came out with the full gamut of gynaecological disorders that could explain the pain. And he went down each rabbit hole with us as a teaching exercise. How would they investigate for these? How would they manage what we found?

"But," he then said, as a kind of finale, "this is what this woman really needs!' And he raised his right arm, flexed at the elbow, fist upright and with his left hand clasped his now tense right biceps all in one rapid movement. We recognised this as the sign of sexual intent on behalf of a man: "That is what will fix her complaint!"

Now it became apparent to me about the skill of the man and his interview techniques. It did mean he had a challenge in front of them with the couple, although I suspect it was consummately managed.

When I was later to become a resident in psychiatry, and about the time the young woman with the overdose died in front of me, I came upon an American visiting psychiatrist called Bob who was remarkable in being able to elicit psychological problems with his interview technique, and also to get his patient to look the problem square in the face.

Apart from the sexist implications of the story, which did after all get the point across quite succinctly, was the deep impression that these men – and women on occasion – made on me. I was to become impressed about the interview process, the value of the patient's story, and respect for their values and beliefs.

An interesting aside was that this same gynaecological consultant had written a paper in the defining medical student textbook on gynaecology. I went back to it and scanned it from cover to cover. Nowhere in it was there anything like the story he had told. But, maybe more significantly, nowhere was there anything about the relationship of sexuality to gynaecological disorders. In hindsight, I could see that this education was not absent, it was simply reserved for the kind of teaching encounter I am illustrating here. This is more a true apprenticeship, I reasoned.

I was more than a little reflective. Kennan's recent stories from his training days were entirely about medicine as an art; he had obviously not considered it either relevant or appropriate to provide ones more scientific or technical. There would be some, of course, but Kennan's explanation was that they didn't demonstrate what medicine has lost, being the art and practice of medicine as a tradition with an apprenticeship component.

Yet the nature of the stories was also interesting. As indicated, I was beginning to understand that the alcohol aspect of some of the stories related at least to Kennan's more recent experiences, and that recounting them was possibly as much therapeutic to him as instructive to others. But did this really matter? Was I a scribe to his story or a counselling facilitator; a healer of sorts for the healer? Then I realised I was circulating around and repeating some of my earlier reflections of hidden motives in his account. I started to look at him judgmentally as I reflected, but received a blank look in return. Did he know what I was thinking?

Less personal maybe was that the content of the stories had a death component; you'd expect that in medicine, of course. Yet they were also significantly focused on birth and sex. I have already related the concern about the loss of relationship of sexuality to health in western medicine, but I was beginning to discern how a deeper pattern or cycle – of birth, sex and death

– was permeating the stories as well as the account as a whole.

We paused. I was again very reflective: I wondered why after all this rich experience that Kennan had subsequently decided on surgery as a career? He felt that it seemed easy now to recount these stories as if he had an understanding of the various depths and dimensions present in them, but at the time of occurrence he did not. In fact, it was because he found these potential depths almost overwhelming that he wanted to do something in medicine that was practical and purposeful.

This implied there was much that was not purposeful. Kennan agreed. He felt that much was done in medicine for the wrong reasons and that many of the premises on which management were based were also incorrect. I asked for examples in each category and he went straight for the jugular.

"Well, we often do pathology and other investigations for the wrong reasons. We do this because we believe if we can find disease before symptoms emerge or physical signs reveal to us, then there is a greater chance of cure. But the facts do not bear this out. In fact, we get into more of a mess with so-called early detection as well as catering to people's fears, often leaving them worse off. It's the fears we should be addressing directly and not exploiting them.

"I also have little doubt that we have the wrong view of the causes of cancer. Because we base our treatment on the cause and when it doesn't work, why don't we then go back and ask ourselves whether we have it right? We don't with cancer."

"So, what do you think causes cancer?" I asked, but not disagreeing with anything he had said to date, although I was careful to avoid showing it.

"I don't think it is a question of a cause, I think it is more a manifestation." Now he had my attention. "I suspect that things go amiss beyond the physical – in the metaphysical – and unless they are corrected at that level, then they manifest physically."

"Are you talking about psychosomatic medicine?"

"That's too simplistic because it looks at the problem from the physical point of view – soma – rather than the metaphysical – psyche. It may also be too early to discuss this all in any meaningful way. Let's get on with the account and see where we go."

He was quite abrupt. I was a little started, as this was a side of him I had not previously seen.

I could see now how the stories from London were so significant, and also how they would have been to someone of Kennan's disposition. But, at the time he heard them, they had almost overwhelmed, or maybe frightened him with their implications, and pushed him into the realms of the practical with surgery. Although the questions may have seemed too big at the time, they obviously affected him and were even to lead him away from a surgical career when the doors were opening in that direction in a beckoning manner.

Three

Beyond the concerns and some moderate confusion that I might have been entertaining about Kennan at a personal level, I was professionally able to resonate with much that he recounted to me. My stories from my rather too frequent and extensive interactions with medicine were different and maybe not as colourful or insightful, but there was a similarity in the themes, even though only from the perspective of a recipient. This could easily be reflective of our similar dispositions, but I suspect there is more to it than this. Why, for example, was he not recalling stories focused on the amazing technological and pharmaceutical advances that paralleled his career? This had been the sort of material that had formed much of my writing about medicine; that was, until I met Kennan.

When I asked him this, I received, in return, a long period of reflection. Now that I had pointed this out, Kennan told me he found it interesting as well. Maybe it was because we were and are still in the phase of appreciating the significance of these advances from a more ethical perspective, and that we still had a way to go in this venture. Irrespective, he did feel that medical science was over-exclusive and relatively dismissive of other approaches and disciplines. He also felt that technology was relied on too much and not used in the right manner or context, all too frequently. But more likely it was because his stories contained truths and wisdom that we might be lacking in medical conversation, need to reconnect to, and be required in today's overly technological climate to further the ethical debate. Was he being arrogant, or simply objectively truthful?

Before we explored what these stories may represent, Kennan reflected on stories generally and his personal narrative in particular. He likened them to myths and other collective tales that held wisdom, which would become relevant at times in our evolution when such wisdom was lacking in the present. And mythology or narrative does this in a symbolic form that appeals more deeply to us, circumnavigating our cognitive resistance or conditioning that can inhibit our listening to any inconvenient truth. So, trusting that remembering tales like this were not simply his disposition or even personal prejudice, but was also a recollection of things that may be or become important, both personally and collectively. In this I could see that he saw himself as more a vehicle or channel in his story-telling. My concern about his arrogance took another dent.

Kennan then started to look at what we had covered so far from his understanding of them. Most obvious in the stories to date is the perspective and position of the patient and his or her practitioner. As he gained experience, he recognised that this significance was because they contained other health features the modern scientific orientation tended to exclude. From the patient's perspective, this involves respecting their attitudes, beliefs and values. From a more patient-centred practitioner viewpoint, it is their mental outlook, cognitive framework, and emotional or even spiritual life.

Kennan then elaborated verbatim: "Modern medicine is wrestling with this balance somewhat awkwardly, by including psychiatry as a specialty compatible with others in medicine, which it definitively is not. Medicine has also annexed psychology as a discipline, but has limited this inclusion to the academic, research and strictly clinical dimensions – that is, mainly the cognitive and behavioural ones, largely excluding anything emotional or spiritual – rather like the acceptance of certain alternative health care practices under the title

Complementary Medicine within mainstream medicine. This inclusion is under the terms of the medical establishment and their defining criteria, and is certainly not holistic.

"There are also other perspectives of health in the world. The social setting has been defined as important in medicine by the WHO in 1949, but since only tacitly included, if at all. This had been the case with the dock worker mentioned earlier, where if the aspiring doctor's premature view of his social circumstances had been taken on board, then the man would have been labelled with an unnecessary disease diagnosis and boosting statistics. There is far too much of this in modern medicine.

"That this social dimension includes family and ancestral networks is maybe appreciated to a limited and mundane extent in medical genetics, but not in its wider mythic and spiritual ramifications. One only needs to look at generational trauma to recognise this. The environment has been ignored to our peril, and not just with such issues as climate change, but also with nutrition and such concerns as the pervasiveness of pharmaceuticals."

Some or all of these features Kennan had embedded in his stories to date, and they would emerge into a more holistic medical and worldview he was to maintain for many years in the latter part of his career and beyond. But he put more stress on the actual relationship of the patient and doctor, as this contains a dynamic that was essential to any genuine healing, rather than mere symptomatic treatment. He also, and controversially, sees this to include or be mainly erotic in nature.

Yet more than this, and as illustrated in the story of the Atlantic rower, it was about the relationship of patients with themselves. If this relationship manifested through problems with health, then the further relationship with the doctor was essential in restoring any loss or deficiency. Kennan also considered that it was the breakdown of the relationship patients had with themselves that stood behind much illness and disease. I could recognise the spectre of issues like stress and trauma here and their significance.

Was this where the priest should be present, but is no more? Has our loss of connection to our spirituality with the dominance of science ruptured this connection and – ironically – created much in the way of distress and disease? Is psychology a poor substitute for this and the so-called new age an attempt to restore it? Are the alternative and complementary health disciplines a return of this to restore a balance to mainstream?

These questions would remain hanging in the air for a while. Instead, Kennan was to focus on the question of responsibility, because, up to this point in our narrative, the stories had been witnessed by him as a kind of passive observer. With qualification as a doctor and acceptance as a probationary or pre-registration medical practitioner he started to experience the weight of responsibility, and his stories started to reflect this more acutely, so back to his account.

> Toward the end of my medical training in London there was an opportunity for mature students to undertake an apprenticeship of sorts. Should a qualified probationary resident in a hospital find it difficult to find a replacement – called a locum – for a holiday or break, then a senior medical student might be invited to fill the position. Effectively, and for this period, the student behaved and was treated like a qualified doctor and probationary practitioner.
>
> I had come to know a neighbouring hospital in the city of Colchester quite well with student secondments. I was invited to fill a resident role there and subsequently did several posts, as I found the experience invaluable. I was also counselled that

dealing with the final medical examinations was easier with this sort of practical experience.

Colchester was a rich and sometimes overwhelming experience for me. Most of my time was as a locum surgical resident. I can see this exposure now as being pivotal in my subsequent choice to pursue surgery as a career, because at Colchester, after the rigours of training, I found myself as an accepted part of a team with a very practical and seemingly effective outlook.

Although the responsibility was relative – I always had someone to 'sign off' on what I had decided and was doing – it was a step into practice and effectively no different from being a qualified pre-registration resident. In many ways, I was an apprentice in the true sense of the word. And this included an antiquated roster system that was significant in my choice to move to Australia after qualifying. This was the 1-in-3, or 1-in-2 residency that in effect meant that, depending on the position, a resident was on emergency call 33 to 50% of the time, day and night.

My position was a 1-in-2, so I was on call every other night and sometimes two nights in a row, as well as emergency intake during any allotted day. I recall assisting my registrar (a trainee specialist) at an operation when he leaned across the operating table, lifted the surgical instrument out of my hand, and said: "Go to bed!"

I had been up all night and most of the night before. I was literally falling asleep on my feet. This would mean that my registrar would cover me for a while. But that was the nature of the team and the social network in which it was embedded.

It was the same registrar who quizzed me as they were about to start an appendix operation. He simply asked me how to do the operation. I rattled off the technique, presuming he was testing my knowledge, but, when I was halfway through my account, he looked directly at me, handed me the scalpel, and then took over the assistant role. My first appendix operation was conducted as a student; how times have changed.

I also recall the time an alcoholic publican on my ward became delirious some three days after an operation for a burst stomach ulcer. I found him exiting the ward surrounded by various tubes and drips on trolleys, with a number of anxious nurses in his wake. The man was sweating profusely and presumably the pink elephants were having their say. I retired to the tearoom to work out a sedative regime.

"What are you doing?" asked the interested anaesthetist who had put the man to sleep for his original operation. I told him.

"The man is an alcoholic?"

The question was rhetorical, but I answered yes anyway.

"So, use an alcohol drip."

I had never heard of this suggestion, but realised there was alcohol in some of the intravenous drip preparations. So, I replaced an existing drip with this and turned up the flow. The man rapidly became calm and I then turned the flow down. This regime was kept that way for the remainder of the patient's time on the ward. My consultant raised no objection, just a smile. They presumed he would return to his habitual ways minus the burst ulcer on discharge, but were also prepared for his return at some future time with another alcohol-related health problem. They didn't believe they could do any more than they were doing to help him, and I noted other psychological interventions had been tried, but to no avail. It was a practical stance, and resources were not being unnecessarily wasted or unrealistic treatments and cures espoused.

Here I was making choices and decisions and ... acting on them. I was taking responsibility for my patient's welfare. The degree to which this was simply fixing up problems or actually mending patients' problems – and their ways – did not occur to me then, or appeared only marginally in my thinking. But I was certainly experiencing that the practicalities and efficacy of management was often outside the emerging tendency to treat all people with a particular diagnosis according to a strict protocol. I was also to experience the bottom line; the actual all too real limits of my profession in disease management.

As a further example is the farmer who came in with a thumb wound. He had fallen over a fence and his thumb took the brunt of his fall, but he thought little of the dirty wound beneath the nail. When I first saw him, he was already ill and destined to die from tetanus, and in spite of all my decisions and endeavours, I was to witness the limits of science. This saddened me greatly, although was a lesson in its own right.

The farmer had become my friend. Later, as a qualified probationary resident in Perth, I had a similar relationship with a man of forty with a chronic relapsing pancreatic condition. He was a quiet man; little passed between us; but every day I went in to put in a new needle for his intravenous feeding. I ran out of sites for this and, like a drug-addict, I became very imaginative. The man never flinched; we had a silent rapport. He survived the duration of my tenancy on that ward, but died a couple of days after I left. Even then I had a feeling about why he may have died, but because it involved himself subjectively, this remained marginal in my reflections as the implications were too big for me to countenance at the time.

I returned to London enriched by my various experiences at Colchester. My final examinations were a challenge, but I tackled them with confidence, helped by my experiences as an apprentice. The only real challenge for my medical final examination was that the main case I was given to present was a woman with chronic paranoid schizophrenia. I feverishly examined her, aware of the story of the student given a mental health patient who also had multiple sclerosis, but that this had been missed by the student.

I could find nothing on a meticulous physical examination and felt nervous fronting the examiners. Before them I fudged my way through the psychiatric questions, feeling cheated and hard done by. I had incorrectly reasoned that psychiatry would not be part of the clinical case and not studied this accordingly. I was devastated immediately afterwards, but passed. I did not know whether I was given that case because I had – effectively – already done enough to test my abilities to this point. Maybe it was a sign of what was to come. Irrespective, a week later, I was on the plane to Australia.

The story about the publican sparked my interest, for reasons already expressed, but Kennan's account of the farmer and his death made me tearful. We discussed the management and its failure in some detail, almost as colleague to colleague, but the way the farmer's story had affected me did not escape his notice. Was he also teaching me, I began to wonder?

The difference between learning to be a practitioner and actually being one would seem to be one of linear progress, with the final examination to qualify as a medical doctor some sort of rite of passage. Yet whilst it is an initiation, it is much more. It is a transition from simply observing a patient and their situation and coming to some sort of judgement about their condition, to actually being involved in the process.

This is a huge responsibility. The diagnosis and subsequent choice of management carries all kinds of personal biases depending on the person making it; hence the importance of the pre-registration probationary period. Of course, modern science and technology has tried to get away from this conundrum with all sorts of testing procedures, but to little avail. Also, the establishment of protocols is a misguided attempt to circumvent the inherent human aspect of diagnosis and management, as well as to limit errors.

Pathology and radiological investigations abound, but rather than being used for information they are increasingly used diagnostically, as well as being a way for the practitioner to obviate the personal responsibility in taking a history and conducting an examination. Both Kennan and I consider this a gross error, as it is not what investigations are primarily for. It is also one of the reasons that approaches in medicine, such as testing for disease prior to its manifestation, are not proving effective and even creating further problems.

Why do Kennan and I think this way? Because there is no getting around subjectivity, as it is an inherent part of the process. And ignoring it by trying to place the responsibility onto investigations is fraught with error – as is becoming increasingly evident – and avoids the important role of subjectivity. The clinician who makes the diagnosis is making a judgement, and is intimately involved with the person about whom that judgement is being made. Medicine is an art as well as, if not more than, a science.

Kennan and I also have an interest in physics and we know from the frequently vexing discoveries made in quantum physics that subjectivity cannot be eliminated from an experiment or observation. In fact, there is a view that experimental outcome depends on it or – in the more radical perspective – is actually driven or created by it. If this is indeed the case, and we believe it is, modern medicine with all its objectivity is well out of date. Also, the onus on subjectivity has further implications, even more magical ones.

One medical field that exemplifies this is psychiatry. In spite of attempts to change this fact and claim objectivity, it remains the case that all – *all* – psychiatric diagnoses are subjective. So, seemingly in spite of himself, it was no surprise that, of all the medical disciplines that Kennan was a probationary resident in, psychiatry was to have the most significant effect in that formative year. He has described the influence, even if indirectly, at the very onset of this account. He also rued its interference in his medical finals. But as he struggled to try and make a practical career out of surgery during the course of this formative year, it was the whole domain of the psychological that was to increasingly dominate his view of medicine.

Kennan sat and sipped his coffee, reflecting on his pre-registration. Ironically, apart from one significant story from his posting in psychiatry, and the one about the patient with the relapsing condition he already mentioned, there were none he was drawn to. And, when he considered it, the one about that particular patient was hardly to do with surgery.

Wondering why this was, Kennan came to the conclusion that, by comparison to Colchester, he had by no means the degree of responsibility that engendered relevant stories. The British health system at that time was stressed and undermanned, and that gave trainees like him opportunities he may not otherwise have been exposed to. The irony was that he also left Britain because of this stress and prospects of his long-term professional future. He was married, his wife was pregnant, so he also had a family to consider now.

Australia, by contrast, had a fundamentally different – private – health system, so that the public system where he did his registration residency was less busy and stressed than its British equivalent. The future in private medicine looked good, but the path to it provided less experience than Kennan would otherwise have obtained in Britain. Maybe he should have stayed in Britain. Indeed, many trainee specialists went there purely for the experience they would get in the overburdened National Health System.

As a consequence, by comparison to Colchester and hence Britain generally, his residency year for registration was a breeze. The registrars were grabbing any of the work, and hence decision-making. The resident picked up the pieces, followed direction, and was more of a glorified scribe. With a baby and family, this situation suited Kennan at the time, but was to change dramatically when he became medically registered and undertook a post in Kalgoorlie, in regional Western Australia.

But before he recounted this, Kennan told me there was one story from his psychiatric residency posting that had a deep impression on him. Not only did it change his perspective about responsibility in health, it also contained the seeds of his future interests in psychotherapy. This was also because generally psychiatry in Australia was relatively 'organic' – it had a primarily physical, mechanical, and pharmaceutical orientation … and still does. By contrast, elsewhere in the world there was often more of an emphasis on the branch called 'dynamic' psychiatry, which was more psychotherapeutically inclined.

This was the emphasis of the visiting professor of psychiatry from America. He conducted his teaching by interviewing a patient in front of his students. In general patients were usually 'talked about' in clinical meetings that did not include them, or only if it was clinically appropriate. This particular professor – Bob, who we briefly came across in the preceding chapter – did not have the same sensibility.

I recall his interview technique. On this occasion, Bob had outlined the patient's problem prior, and to all intent and purposes it was distinctly neurotic – meaning that he did not have a formal diagnostic psychiatric disease like schizophrenia, but was experiencing anxiety about life conflicts and choices that he was not facing. As this seemed to be the bulk of the sort of patient that came to a psychiatrist, it was probably no surprise that my initial reactions to psychiatry were of disinterest.

Bob sat in front of the patient and quite close, the students somewhat more distant. So, there was a zone of sorts that separated doctor and patient from the onlookers. Bob, previously unknown to the patient, introduced himself and the purpose of the interview that included the students' presence. With the patient's agreement, the interview then proceeded.

All this was of no surprise to me, although I did wonder why Bob had chosen such a boring case. Once Bob had outlined the problem, he then asked the patient if he agreed with Bob's assessment. He did. Then Bob proceeded to probe with more questions that patiently, subtly and cleverly unravelled the unspoken psychological patterns in the patient's position. Periodically came a similar request for agreement from the patient, or at least acknowledgement of Bob's proposed possible reasoning contained in the question.

By this stage I was engrossed. This was more forensic in nature and appealed to me, like a good detective story. In fact, there were many similarities, which further attracted my attention. Eventually it seemed that Bob had taken a circuitous route that evaded the patient's normal rational defences to his problem, led him right to it, and then culminated with the "do you agree?" question in such a manner that the patient could only agree with Bob. The alternative would have been for the patient to hit him, so complete was the exposure and so close was Bob ... almost inviting it.

I was impressed. Impressed to the point that he took time out to watch further interviews by Bob and also to engage with him personally, as well as in his other clinical and teaching activities. It seemed to me that Bob had confronted the patient with the source of his problem in such a way that he was obliged to accept and, most importantly, take responsibility for it.

I was later to find out that this approach had a philosophical nature about it. Plato, some 2,500 years before, had Socrates as his written mouthpiece undertake similar lines of questioning to express his own point of view. Yet the fact that it did draw on philosophy was intriguing, as this was a discipline that he would not otherwise have been exposed to. A surprise I considered in my later years, as it had and has much to offer psychology and psychiatry, yet remains relatively ignored.

The regional hospital post at Kalgoorlie represented many challenges. When I realised I'd been given poor post-registration residency posts because of my decision to train as a surgeon but then withdrawing, my reaction was to return the favour. I surreptitiously approached the State Health Department and applied for a regional post. I was provisionally given a more attractive, interesting and autonomous position in the Kimberley.

But this was not without knowing that my first residency post was regional, where I knew I would get a lot of practical experience. Now registered, I accepted the second-year postings given to me, knowing full well that I would tender my resignation at the end of the first posting when the Health Department job became available. At least, that was the plan. Circumstances would dictate otherwise ...

The posting was six hundred kilometres from State's capital of Perth, and I drove there with my wife and our baby daughter. Some two-thirds of the way there, we were held up by a sandstorm. We had not seen or been in anything like this before. It did not bode well, particularly with the drive after this point that felt like a one-way journey into a desert. By contrast, when we finally arrived, the regional city seemed like an oasis; although more like Las Vegas than the tropical equivalent.

The reason I had taken this post was that this large mining town of Kalgoorlie had an interesting medical structure at that time. It was effectively run by the general practitioners, as was the hospital. I was one of three residents, so there was a 1-in-3 roster and the local doctors were more than happy for we residents to take on as much work as we could or felt capable of and then they providing the backing, if necessary. So, the roster was not as rigid as my days in England and I could also live at home nearby when on call, because a great deal could be managed by phone.

There were three specialists there, as I recall now. But they were only involved if either the local general practitioner or resident referred to them. Alternatively, there was the Royal Flying Doctor service and Perth. All in all, this was quite a different set up to what I had experienced to date, with ample latitude depending on temperament. It also symbolically matched the town, as it was effectively the Wild West, as I was soon to discover!

There were more stories here than I care to mention. There was also a significant and itinerant aboriginal population that added a particular richness to medical practice. I found this out one day when I was asked by the Police to certify the death of a man found in the bush. When the constable pointed to the rear of the utility vehicle with a smile on his face, I knew I had something coming. And I did, although I was forewarned by the stench. I pulled back the cover to reveal an old aboriginal man who had obviously been dead for several weeks!

I also delivered a syphilitic baby in the back of a plane with my bare hands. The aboriginal mother delivered as soon as I climbed in and I effectively caught a near moribund child. The state of the afterbirth confirmed my suspicions. An embarrassed locum flying doctor, who had not felt emotionally equipped to handle the situation, looked on silently with a pale face.

The baby quietly died, assisted by my non-intervention in the ambulance on the way to the hospital, and the mother simply gazed out of the window. She knew. What was more distressing for me was to see the covering general practitioner become convinced that he could hear a faint heartbeat and try to revive the baby once we arrived at the hospital. After a bit of reflection, I decided to have two big injections of penicillin in his bum. Just in case.

I had already seen enough death. If my days on the farm had not already primed me, one of the postings in the casualty department whilst a resident had given me more. Because of my reputation for practicality and not being phased by almost anything that came across my path, I was often positioned in the resuscitation unit. In a casualty department that is the emergency hub of a city at that time, there isn't much you don't see.

Gold mining was the main industry of Kalgoorlie. There is a lot of gambling, drinking and women; one street was lined with brothels. As a married man, I knew I had to limit my social scope. I was not a gambler anyway, but drinking had to be closely watched, as I could detect my own potential future concerns in some older colleagues. Illicit drugs were also on offer, but as I had already seen the risks in the contents of the doctor's bag in others and having a social and therapeutic relationship with alcohol, I decided that this was not a path I wanted to go on, even though the knowledge of hallucinogens and their effects intrigued me at the time. I was also more socially adventurous than my two resident colleagues, so spent my time with the local doctors and their families.

As my rostered posting drew to a close, I was contacted with the anticipated letter from the Health Department about the posting I had received. At the same time, and completely out of the blue, I received a call from one of the local doctors, who was also the busiest practitioner in town. Stewart had just lost his infant child after a short illness. He and his wife were devastated and he decided to take six months off, if possible. Stewart rang me offering a locum to run his private practice.

I was flabbergasted, as I had also been offered a general practice position in a successful Perth general practice for some time in the near future, and the timing for this was open. The partners there wanted me as a future partner, but also appreciated that I may need a bit more experience, which they believed my anticipated Health Department position would provide; but this post was a minimum of one year, and that seemed too long in the overall timing. I discussed the locum option that Stewart offered with the partners, who saw a distinct advantage in it. So, I resigned from my present rotational posting, declined the Health Department's post, and stepped into private general practice.

The decisions here seemed rapid, I remarked to Kennan. "They were," he replied, blaming the carefree style of the town, although I viewed it also as his nature. Later he was to tell me about an affair with the wife of one of the high school teachers there, known or even condoned by him; they were West Coast American, after all! When I would have thought that would have complicated things even further, Kennan somehow implied the reverse and that it clarified things for him. I wasn't sure whether this was a difference of moral position between us, but let that thought pass. I was not surprised that his marriage, born of Oxford and middle-class England, was not to survive much longer.

But why choose general practice?

Kennan explained that it was a kind of marking time. It gave him some space to look at his marriage in comfortable circumstances and less high-paced pressure. It also did not close the door on specialisation into the future; he just needed a breather. Also, maybe the scope of a general practice, like the one he would step into in Perth, would help him make future decisions of this kind. After all, the Perth practice did their own obstetrics, minor surgery, and anaesthetics in addition to consulting. Yet, for all the busyness of the locum and the many memories Kennan has, one story stood out and would – again – point to his future.

> It was a very, very busy day at the surgery. The nurse had sequestered a mother and infant in a corner of her treatment room. The child, about a year old, had a temperature that the nurse thought was insignificant. I passed by the door and the nurse clutched me, anxious to lighten the heavy patient load by one. I checked the child and found nothing wrong. As I came out with the usual verbal patter of "I can't find anything wrong, but take some paracetamol and if things change or get worse … blah blah."
>
> I felt awkward. Instinctively I knew there was something wrong, but I didn't know what. So, the rhetoric changed to "I can't find anything wrong, but I am not comfortable with his condition … do you mind if we admit him to the ward overnight for observation?"
>
> At midnight, I was called to a very sick child with a rigid neck and unable to tolerate the light. It was meningitis – a lumbar puncture confirmed this with pus coming out, and the child was on the plane to the city.
>
> How had I known that? There are many explanations, but ultimately it was intuition to my

mind then, although maybe not now. Yet it wasn't that simple. I was vulnerable at the time with an unsure marriage, so had my emotional state and vulnerability contributed? Did I have a sense of the future with what I somehow saw in this child? And how much did this remind me of the young woman with the overdose who died at the end of my hand?

More questions than answers. Again. Shortly afterwards, the family packed their bags and returned to Perth when the locum finished. Life – and his marriage – would start anew with a house on the hill overlooking a lake, and a position as the partner in a bustling and successful general practice down the road. Was this Kennan's future?

Four

I made a decision to write this chapter of Kennan's three years' experience within general practice in the third person. This was mainly because I felt that his narrative during this period led to conclusions with which I could readily resonate to and agree with. So, they are views and positions that are common to both of us; although Kennan's understanding, born of direct experience, preceded my similar realisations by many years.

The decision was also because there would otherwise be too many stories. I had gravitated to putting the stories directly into Kennan's mouth when I committed them to writing. With so many during this period, I felt the need to edit and condense these into some general conclusions with which we were both comfortable. My experience of this period was one of harmony and ease, our relationship had moved to a common position in spite of any misgivings or concerns I may have had about him as a person.

One discussion that Kennan and I have had over the years, and have frequently returned to, is the current state of the health system in Australia. Ironically, the public system that was in such disarray when he left Britain several decades ago now seems a better option than the current private one in Australia, which is quite dysfunctional, open to abuse and even fraud. In Kennan's terms, the current health system is "bankrupt, insane and very scary." I would also point out that these remarks – in fact all this chapter – were made and committed to writing well before the Covid pandemic of 2020, which has only served to highlight many of his and my concerns, and to which we will come.

We even played a 'mind game' of sorts: What would happen if Medicare and all health insurance, including pharmaceutical cover, were no longer available? Although we had some fun with what might occur to the various institutions and policing agencies that had grown up around health and medicine – what Kennan refers to as the Medical Industrial Complex – this was tempered by the social implications of such a change. Yet this was simply a mind game, one you can follow to see where it takes you, and sometimes with surprising results. Our thinking went in various directions, so here are some of the outcomes; it is specifically targeted at the medical establishment.

Would there be a more exaggerated two-tier health system, with the 'haves' having access to services and the 'have-nots' relatively excluded? Or would the 'haves' look more deeply at their position and explore alternatives in healthcare delivery, depending on the real evidence of its success, and consider the 'have-nots' in this process?

Would doctors then be selected for their innate skills, including the once-lauded 'bedside manner'? And would this mean that their fees would reflect their abilities and success more directly? Would this lead to an undercurrent of 'keeping people well', rather like the veterinarian, and would we see the resurrection of more traditional approaches like 'folk' medicine, rather like the so-called barefoot doctors of China?

Counselling, education and mentoring may take an increased role in the management of illness and disease. This could lead to a greater sense of self-responsibility and hence self-health management, which I am aware Kennan believes is the foundation of any future change in the health system.

With the expense of pharmaceuticals, would we question their necessity, as well as realise and rediscover that there may be an equivalent herb for every ailment? Would we then pay more attention to nutrition and exercise, and inculcate it within the youth at a family level? Would prevention then take on a greater, and maybe more holistic and genuine role than it does at present?

What about all the surgery? All the repairs, corrections, and myriad so-called apparently 'needless' operations: Would these diminish? Would we consider a hip or knee prosthesis quite so quickly, or might we try remedial methods first and even actively promote preventative ones prior?

And all the investigations that we have, which may not help us but simply instill more fear and illness behaviour: Would we begin to question what they achieve, maybe more than we do presently? Would we consider a cup of tea and a held hand as an alternative to an analgesic? Might we reconsider the role of topical treatments such as poultices and ointments?

Might we seriously – and properly for the first time – take into consideration environmental health issues? These include the poisons in our homes and ones we use in our routine daily habits. Would our cosmetic appearance matter as much if its relationship to our health were fully recognised?

Would alternative and complementary practices, which are probably more equipped than modern medicine for such an alternate eventuality, return to favour? Might we look at the so-called new age healing practices with a bit more seriousness?

Might we get away from what is presented as the lauded evidence-based medicine being the prerogative of mainstream medicine? Would we see it as the Medical Industrial Complex – and specifically the pharmaceutical industry – manipulating data to suit their own agendas? With such evidence as a basis, could we honour the anecdotal and the voice of experience?

Would the evidence start to stack up that we don't need all that excessive and sometimes unnecessary surgery, preventative pharmaceutical treatment, and simple over-servicing that feeds our fears and makes us the 'worried well'?

And what about our trainees: Would students select medicine if they weren't guaranteed an income by Medicare at the end of it? Also, if the social prestige of being a doctor diminishes, would that impact on the demand for medical student places?

As medicine historically draws the most intelligent in our student community into a profession that doesn't demand that level of intelligence, once qualified, would that free up these bright minds for other fields? Might it also reduce the inevitable dissatisfaction that would greet these individuals in the routine and mundaneness of everyday practice?

Where would medicine go if it weren't economically, but also politically, legally and socially regulated? Would doctors once more gain autonomy and public trust, as well as be free to practice their art, take risks, and become once again the practitioners of old with the associated respect that has all but gone in the modern era?

In summary: Will we come to the conclusion that modern western medicine is good in the case of an accident or an emergency, but beyond that be an expensive and largely unnecessary luxury?

The questions mount up. Each one takes us down a rabbit hole and might – would – lead us to unexpected outcomes. But how can that be the case, asked Kennan and myself; how did we get to this "bankrupt, insane and very scary" state, and what is the solution?

Kennan, of course, had some answers, or at least proposals. His belief is that the present health system, including modern western medicine, is close to or even beyond the point that it can heal itself. And he certainly believes this is nigh on impossible if the profession itself, or its supporting 'masters', attempt it. Nothing less than a complete change, a paradigm shift, is needed; he believes that is now an inevitable outcome. It is just that whether, rather like any birthing process, it can be managed to minimise complications, or even death in the process.

These sorts of questions had really not crossed Kennan's mind until he joined the general practice partnership. Up until this time he had been salaried in the public sector, or given a fixed wage as a locum. But now, in his own practice, he started to equate each person he saw and what he charged him or her from his hip pocket. But not only that, all the partners did – unashamedly.

The above questions became an evolving part of his reality in this period. Not all at once, of course, but depending on his circumstances, both medically and socially. They are an important part of this account and will evolve in the narrative as it unfolds. The outcome is not that all the above questions are answered; too many of them are either rhetorical, or simply unanswerable. But collectively they lead to a position that both coincides with Kennan's current awareness and also offers a way of dealing with them; a kind of 'walking your talk'.

The first realisation that Kennan had was almost overwhelming: The vast majority of patients who came to see him didn't have a medical problem. Also, even if they did, they commonly did not need his services. How could this be? He was so accustomed to believing that anyone in a doctor's care is sick – why otherwise would you be occupying a bed in a London teaching hospital – that he hadn't been taught the prior question: Is this person actually sick and needing my care in the first place?

Of course, this itself was an evolving question for Kennan, but he recalls that somehow it became more acute when he had his own practice and not someone else's, be it a hospital or as a locum in Stewart's practice. It was somehow connected to the issue of responsibility, although that felt a bit vague at the time.

Yet it caused him to reflect and try and keep some sort of mental record of what it was that brought people to consult him.

The outcome of this was interesting. Kennan considered it a rare week when he made a new diagnosis of a medical disease, as opposed to illness, unwellness, or whatever equivalent term you may want to use. Many came for reassurance, but not all wanted education, some still wanted or needed a script. In a growing community, many mothers brought their children, concerned about these little beings, who were often unable to articulate their distress. The responsibility then seemed to fall on him, where parent education became important.

Of course, many were follow-ups and those seeking repeat scripts. The latter became so voluminous that these were often done without a consultation – for a small fee of course! There were referrals to specialists, often because the general practitioner was now seen as some sort of middleman and no longer had a distinct social role. Increasingly, these referrals were to paramedical practitioners, such as physiotherapists and latterly psychologists.

An attempt has been to address this by affording general practice a specialist status, although neither is fooled that this has changed the status of the general practitioner within the profession or in the eyes of the public; instead, it has added years to post-graduate training and therefore further institutionalization … and indoctrination, adds Kennan, as I write.

Kennan reflected a little and felt that there were two medical patterns in his experience that may help clarify some of the above issues and questions. The first was a feature that he felt overwhelmed with and seriously concerned about: young children who had middle ear infections. In a growing suburban area, there were lots of children. When he started to see the number that had already been treated with multiple courses of antibiotics and subsequently ear surgery, he became concerned and wondered about how he might approach this minor epidemic and see if it was all it appeared to be.

In this, Kennan had not forgotten his own childhood, so this might have been what attracted him to this issue in the first place. It is difficult for him to recall but, in hindsight, he wonders how much of the realisations about his own childhood treatment came as a result of his management and understanding of these children. In other words, that his own wounding helped heal others and hence ultimately himself, as well.

Although he had a lot of personal backtracking to do, he decided to keep the matter simple and make a particular note of new cases. The first presentation was often a mother bringing in a crying child, usually pre-verbal, apparently in pain. In looking for the source of pain, hopefully to reassure Mum that it was a touch of 'colic' or something equally spurious, Kennan would often come across an ear that was red (strictly speaking a red eardrum and commonly representative of the state of the middle ear behind).

If both eardrums were red, Kennan often reasoned that this might be the crying itself, which then begged the question of why the child was crying in the first place and would often change the subsequent course of the consultation. Alternatively, it may be just one ear, and this concerned him a little more. What he decided to do in such cases, reasoning that no harm would come to the child in the short term, was to ask Mum to use an analgesic, if necessary, and return the next day so that he could examine the ear or ears again, with no additional charge to Mum.

Actually, he charged a Medicare refund or bulk-billed, and so raised some of the other questions in our list above, including one only briefly touched upon; that of 'over-servicing'. In our earlier mind game, we already knew that over-servicing would greatly diminish, both because the practitioner would not be able to so easily justify the additional consultation (or procedure), and also because the patient would be more discerning and critical of its requirement in their management.

Kennan considered this was reasonable and justified in this situation. He just hoped he wouldn't have to argue his position; he believed that the results would speak for themselves and justify this approach. Actually, he was later to find this is not how over-servicing is assessed, which somewhat shocked him as he thought positive outcomes would automatically be considered, rather than comparison to a statistical average irrespective of the outcome. Maybe he was just naïve ...

Although the comment about naïveté was a bit of a throwaway one on Kennan's part, I was increasingly impressed about it as a significant moral component of his character. Not only did my aforementioned concerns about a personality disorder in the man continue to diminish, I could see why he was drawn into the drama that led to his leaving medicine – a drama others would have negotiated relatively unscathed.

Anyway, naïve or not, this is how he persisted. What he found was that commonly, even usually, the ear or ears returned to normal the next day. He felt vindicated. On the occasion where this was not the case, and where the child remained distressed, he then used an antibiotic. But he felt relieved that the number that he was committing to antibiotic treatment, and maybe future surgery at such an early age, was significantly reduced.

Now Kennan started to see the pattern in hindsight. A child has a red ear or ears and an antibiotic is given. This, for some reason, becomes repetitive and then the antibiotics 'don't work'. Then the surgeon comes in and puts in a drainage tube for the fluid that accumulates and could lead to initially temporary, but later permanent hearing impairment. Even the surgical procedure can be repetitive and the use of antibiotics rampant.

In many cases, Kennan felt he had broken the cycle, but he

had to ask why they were getting infections in the first place. Even at that early stage of his career, he knew that diet was an issue. Excessive milk and wheat products are strongly implicated, even if the child was not clinically allergic to them. Then he found out about yeast (or candida) and surmised that many of these children get fluid accumulation, or glue ear, because they have yeast infections as a result of the antibiotics, and that sugars (or simple carbohydrates) in the diet are what yeast feeds on.

Medicalisation "is the process by which human conditions and problems come to be defined and treated as medical conditions, and thus become the subject of medical study, diagnosis, prevention, or treatment (definition)". However, and this is the more popular and urban definition: Medicalisation is when illness patterns are managed by medicine in a such way as to create problems that require the same profession to solve them. That is, the process is self-serving.

Medicalisation could be seen as a more subtle, yet pernicious and concerning form of over-servicing. The patterns are too deep or well justified, and sometimes exist because of the exclusion of other diagnostic possibilities (yeast and ear infections), or simpler often non-medical methods of management. Kennan could then begin to see the pattern of medicalization, and it concerned him. He also started to see it elsewhere in his practice and those of his colleagues. But he also found that they either did not or did not want to know.

Hugh was, in most respects, a good diagnostician and doctor. He had a pleasing manner that bordered on the charming, particularly for his female patients, supported by his good looks and athletic build. Kennan learned a lot from him and enjoyed the relationship until a pattern emerged that started to concern him.

This first became obvious on Kennan's rostered work in the partnership. The partners commonly assisted in the operations of patients they had referred. This was by a token invitation from the specialist, as the assistant received a fee for his or her service in the private sector. He found himself frequently assisting the gynaecologist they routinely used, and he became aware that a high proportion of women having hysterectomies were Hugh's patients.

When he then encountered these patients in a consultation, frequently only because Hugh was away on leave, he could start to detect a pattern in their medical history. Often Hugh had first started to see them as teenagers and been involved in contraceptive prescriptions. Inevitably, and in that era, this was the oral contraceptive pill.

Then the patient would marry, go off the pill, and Hugh would deliver the children. Next, after childrearing had finished, he would perform a surgical sterilisation procedure that is now out of date. It requires making a small cut and then going into the body to isolate and block the tubes that bear the eggs by taking a segment of them out. Obviously, this has been superseded over time.

Then the patient would commonly start to get menstrual irregularities of various forms and with varying diagnoses. So, hysterectomy was often the consequence, even if only relatively justified for symptomatic relief. Following this, the patient would pass through menopause, sometimes prematurely because all this intervention for various reasons, and hormone replacement therapy was prescribed.

Of course, at the time the justification for this was manifold. It is but one of countless examples of a medical or surgical management that was a good idea at the time, backed by seemingly solid evidence, but then either becoming superseded or discovered to be a problem. Such is the case with hormone replacement therapy. It is difficult to know how many of the breast cancer patients in their practice, which were then also often assisted at when operated on, were also a result of this medicalisation process.

Hugh was not being negligent; he had a genuine if somewhat restricted belief in what he was doing professionally. And even whilst Kennan was assisting at a hysterectomy, the next generation was being put on the pill back at the surgery. Does this imply the pill is also a concern in this process? The jury is still out, but Kennan is of no doubt that it is.

This is the sort of outline that he and I would then put through the intellectual sieve of our mind game. Our concern was how many boxes it ticked and the motives for this. Of course, most can be – and continue to be – readily justified by the profession with their use of evidence-based medicine. Kennan would have more to say about such apparent evidence later, but even at this stage of his career, this justification concerned him.

We have both noted that such so-called evidence, when seemingly a justification and ignoring other ways of looking at the medical problem, continues to be in the direction of concern. One has only to look in detail at the pharmaceutical industry to see that particular pattern.

In clinical practice, it seemed to Kennan that most patients came not for a physical reason, but because they were emotionally driven for some reason, about which they were usually unaware. His concerns about medicalisation, and hence the direction that physical medicine was taking – including surgery and his previous attraction to it – was an ongoing source of discomfort to him.

As this process was revealing itself to him, both within practice and also in his reflections about it, Kennan's appreciation of why patients came to a doctor started to gain momentum. He started to see that there were psychological undercurrents to a lot of the illness and even disease he saw. But he also started to notice that illness was actually used to see a doctor for other reasons.

Then the penny dropped. How could they do otherwise? How do you come into a doctor and say: "There's actually nothing wrong with me, but I am distraught about the way my teenage son yelled at me this morning." Of course, that could be seen as a justification, if put in the psychological category, but patients fear emotionality being interpreted as having a psychiatric disorder. So, this begs the question of how much in the way of 'psychosomatic disorder' there actually is, and how much the medical system creates it.

This is compounded by the fact that, in theory at that time, a practitioner should not claim a rebate from Medicare for a consultation that is not about a medical problem. Even though psychiatry would seem to be a discipline that justifies and includes emotional presentations, in practice it rarely does. And this is not only because of the patient; it is also because the doctor is usually poorly equipped in this area, both professionally and personally. Note that here is another pathway to medicalisation, increasingly so in the present era, where a psychiatric diagnosis has become a perverse means of empowerment.

If Kennan were to look back at his exposure to psychiatry at that time, the pattern would become clear. In general, he had seen psychiatry as an inconvenience in his endeavour to gain a command of physical medicine. This was also true of practitioners in general. Most do not train in medicine because they are interested in the mind and its workings, which is maybe one reason they almost exclusively treat mental disorders as brain disturbances.

Kennan's prior exposure to psychological medicine generally, and psychiatry specifically, was not totally suppressed. It had a significant impact on him and started now to manifest in his general practice, causing him to adjust his approach. Yet it was the changes that occurred in his personal life that also added to this adjustment.

After the affair in Kalgoorlie, Kennan returned to Perth and did his best to reconstitute his marriage. Just as he felt he was settling into some sort of stability and rhythm, a package arrived from the lady concerned. He was anxious but relieved that it only contained a book by the British existential philosopher Colin Wilson, called *The Outsider*. For the first time in his life, Kennan felt he was in the company of people who saw the world as he did. The book was her personal copy. She obviously trusted he would return it, possibly for a reprise, but she felt he should read it because he "needed to wake up" (her words), which she might be able to determine with the greater experience of her five extra years of age.

Shortly after this, Kennan's marriage ended when he fell in love for the first time in his life. This new relationship was to open him up to his emotional and sexual life, and its associated turbulence, in a way he had not experienced before. His medical practice formed some sort of stable platform during this period, although it was inevitable that his personal life would start to impact on his work.

The turbulence and a series of seemingly coincidental experiences put him in touch with a Jungian analyst. Kennan felt he needed help and support but, like his patients of that time, he did not like the idea of seeing a psychiatrist and being diagnosed as depressed and prescribed to. Alternatively, he felt he had to explore his experience more deeply, and understand where the mood changes and emotional eruptions were taking him.

The analyst Kennan subsequently saw was a follower of the

psychiatrist and depth psychologist Carl Jung, a pupil of Freud, who subsequently carved his own career and approach to mental experience distinct from his mentor. Jung appealed to Kennan, as it had to the author Hermann Hesse, one of the authors described in *The Outsider*, who had also undergone a Jungian analysis. Kennan started therapy sessions that were to lead him into a direction separate from medicine, but in his view, not incompatible with it.

Kennan's attitude to analysis, as a supposedly deeper form of psychotherapy, was that it was for his own personal benefit. He found the more psychospiritual orientation in Jung's approach to be a challenge and to open up lines of personal inquiry he had not previously seen or experienced, even with all his intellectual contacts. In particular, working with his dreams and a journal were of importance to him, and his personal direction from that point on has continued to be so.

Although Kennan revealed more to me about the impact of the affair and what it meant to him, he was hesitant about how much should enter our account. He was comfortable with the above; it was a necessary inclusion, mainly because it had a context for and referred back to his professional life. It was in keeping with his original injunction to me about his personal life, but somewhat relatively … and only just. It is also one reason I have written this section in the third person, otherwise, there would have been even less input of these personal features.

That this position would change over the progression in time of his professional life, as well as in the context of our relationship, is quite important.

The impact on Kennan's practice was significant. He started to better recognise the psychological undercurrents in his patients' presentations, physical or otherwise. And by psychological, he did not restrict this to the purely mental or cognitive, but also appreciated the emotional and even spiritual domains. In fact, he became concerned at the restricted mental view that psychiatry and psychology took, being essentially cognitive, as he experienced the more emotional undercurrents in his patients' turmoil to be of greater significance.

Indeed, Kennan connected this emotional domain to the instinctual and hence sexual – obviously reflecting his own experience at that time – extending to the stress phenomenon and all sorts of distress states, like anxiety, as well as trauma. He also started to connect this with other bodily systems that, in his opinion, modern medicine did and still does not generally deal with well.

Kennan surmised this was because they could not be organically and mechanically well-defined. These included the immune and hormonal systems and would extend to the brain that he would eventually see in this more fluid manner – unlike psychiatry – and even the emerging field of neuroscience. The connection between brain and mind he saw in the more enigmatic and complicated problematic realm of 'consciousness', which he considered a fundamental.

However, these views would only emerge over time, so how did he apply this perspective to practice?

Kennan explained that it involved a perspective shift to the psychological and that this often meant engaging that area with the patient before honing in on the problem. He also recalled his teachers in his training and how they often naturally took such an orientation. In essence, it was looking for deeper or hidden causes or patterns and dealing with them, rather than on symptom management at the manifest level.

As his views were emergent, so was his approach; and it is only now – following the completion of his medical career – that they have gained some sort of harmony and unity. As we will discover, he found out that this is probably impossible to achieve in mainstream practice at the present time.

Although he had not wanted to engage with his therapeutic analysis for anything apart from personal reasons, the experience effectively encompassed Kennan. By using his new approach, patients in his practice then gravitated to him for a psychological direction. This meant taking on a counselling and even a psychotherapeutic perspective. His consultations increased in length but, from the medical rebate perspective, became less remunerative. His partners recognised this and pointed out that he was contributing less to the collective financial pool they each drew from.

Kennan's new analyst was also a psychiatrist, although retired. This had not been the case with his previous analyst. There is no requirement that someone who trains as a psychoanalyst, of whatever persuasion, also be trained in medicine or psychology. Yet with this new mentor, his analysis seemed to kick up a gear and take him into new psychic territory that engrossed him even more.

His analyst tried to persuade him to train and undertake a career change into psychiatry. This was not to primarily be a psychiatrist, but to have it as an adjunct to a psychoanalytic career embedded in the medical profession at the specialist level. Although not unusual overseas and even common in larger western cities, this would be novel in the region of Australia in which he lived and worked. It would also help promote the Jungian orientation.

Kennan resisted such a change for over a year. However, the increasing pressure in his practice, both from the partners and indirectly from patients, led him in that direction in spite of the freedom and exploration he was experiencing in his personal life. He was having fun socially, but psychiatric training would take him back into hospital practice and the lesser income of the public sector. Also, he would have to move away from his personal playground, a significant factor for a single man!

By the following year, Kennan had relented. He applied and was accepted for psychiatric training and resigned from private general practice. The change would be greater than he had anticipated.

But before we took the leap into the realms of mental health, I asked Kennan why he had not recounted many, if any, individual stories about his time in general practice after he returned to Perth. Instead, he had drawn on some general summaries of issues like the ear infections. For explanation, I will recount his response directly:

"Interesting point, Ian. I hadn't noticed it myself; although in truth, I have given you a smattering; it is you who have decided not to include them! Of course, I can recount many stories and incidents, but I guess, that now I had served an apprenticeship of a kind, any such stories may have become repetitive, or did not have the same impact on me, so I guess they might bore any reader and that was also your conclusion. As I became more experienced, I felt I was trying to make more sense of what I was encountering, looking for themes and patterns.

"In fact, if I think about it, the stories I now recall are more about the mistakes I made. Such as failing to realise the man with acute back pain who was actually having a heart attack, but getting unusual symptoms. There were plenty of diagnostic errors, and some surgical mistakes I made. But the impact was more on me emotionally, recognising that I felt deeply for my patients, and was often racked with feelings of guilt or shame when I got things wrong.

"I guess general practice was also becoming routine, and I was losing some interest. Of course, much of this was quite selfish, as my personal life was quite turbulent and the self-preoccupation of therapy had me in its craw. I was starting to become jaded, a bit mechanical, and losing faith in the increasing protocols that encompassed routine medicine, as well as the lack of the social dimension, and some good old-fashioned humour.

"But essentially, I had served my time. I had gone into general practice to actually mark time until my direction became clearer, which it now was. My focus was more forensic in a way, I was looking beyond the band-aiding of a symptom-based approach, which did not sit well with me, and looking for the deeper issues that were in the patterns I was finding, not simply for and in simple mechanical causes. I was tired of turning imbalance and disturbed physiology into pathology, and the reliance on pharmaceuticals or medical fixes, which seemed not to be working when I looked across longer time periods. I was also finding general medicine itself to be prescriptive, ruled by statistical data disguised as 'evidence', and lacking in stories and the value of experience.

"There is something else though, which I am sure we will return to. I started to see problems in terms of pain and trauma of a more general and often deeper historical nature, as well as to becoming more focused on outcome, or prognosis. This was irrespective of any diagnosis, which I often found was wrong and took the patient and practitioner along an incorrect treatment path. I was taking a much broader and cyclic view of medicine and kind of backfilling as my experience grew. In an indirect way, I wondered whether the inquiry awoken in my own therapeutic analysis would be answered in psychiatry."

I am not sure whether Kennan had answered my question. I gave him the benefit of the doubt and moved with him onto the psychiatric wards.

Five

As I entered the room: "You must be the Trick Cyclist!" was all that greeted me.

The diminutive red-haired young man was sitting cross-legged in the middle of his bed in the Intensive Care Unit of the teaching hospital I was now working in. He had an intravenous drip in one arm and two women sat to the far side. Later I was to find out that one was his mother, the other his sister. The latter was crying. I was confronted; I needed to adopt a position of power, and quickly.

"My ward, ten minutes," I replied, an alternative response to a psychiatric interview; obviously, my unique response to the man's provocation.

"You can't do that!" exclaimed the man.

"Well, it's either that or Graylands."

I turned and left the ward, giving instructions to a dumbfounded nursing sister, who had never seen a psychiatric assessment of less than an hour. I was confident which choice the man would make. Graylands is the psychiatric hospital where patients were sent when admitted for necessary involuntarily assessment and care, as could happen to a mental health patient if a doctor so assessed him. It was a risky but calculated manoeuvre on my part, but not one alien to me.

Kennan and I were meeting at a new café that was quieter, which allowed us more time and reflection. I remarked how his decision to do psychiatry seemed to be the first irrevocable choice he had made in his medical career.

"Yes," he replied. "I suppose that is the case. But the choices from hereon are to become progressively more irrevocable, even to leaving medicine altogether!" He followed this with a cynical laugh; but in spite of any resistance, I could not help but join in with him.

Kennan felt his conviction to train as a psychiatrist had arisen from the analytic process and his analyst's influence. Initially, analysis had been for personal therapeutic reasons; it was only later to transition into training and ultimately to qualification as an analyst. The personal reasons for analysis had somehow led him into a life inquiry of the kind Jung referred to as Individuation. The pursuit of this, and assisting others to do the same, as he discovered in general practice, became a unifying theme in his life; however, and as I portrayed in the previous chapter, it was incompatible with general practice of the kind he was in at the time.

Although Kennan saw that psychiatry was the more pathological end of psychology – that is, mental illness or disease as opposed to emotional distress or mental imbalance – it was an extension of his existing profession. Rightly or wrongly, psychiatry was defined by medicine rather than psychology. Whilst this may be applicable to the branch of psychiatry referred to as 'organic', it seemed that its sibling or the 'dynamic' branch was more naturally associated with psychology, and was further connected by its management practice, which was commonly psychotherapeutic, rather than medical. Irrespective of these sometimes-confusing considerations and the difficulty with his psychiatric preference, he felt that he could carve a career in psychiatry that was principally psychotherapeutic, and even to promote the Jungian orientation and discipline, as was occurring elsewhere overseas.

Although it was principally psychologists who practised psychotherapy in the clinical setting, there were also a good number of psychiatrists who did and do, except at that time none was also trained as an analyst. So, this could be a first for Kennan. But as well, psychotherapy is not confined to psychiatric and psychologically trained practitioners; people from other disciplines could train as analysts and practice psychotherapy. Further, members of the religious professions could be seen as psychotherapists.

Psychotherapy thus has a very wide definition. Even today it remains outside of the direct policing of the medical and psychological disciplines, although the latter has tried in the past to do so in many regions. This freedom is a position that Kennan supports. Not only does he have difficulty with such policing anyway, but he also believes that psychotherapy should remain a wide-ranging inquiry into the mind, soul, or spirit.

Even though I found this clarification a little vague and sometimes confusing, I subsequently considered that any reader would find it even more so. As a consequence, I didn't pursue this clarification any further with Kennan, trusting it may become clearer in the narrative more than in any attempt to do so by description. Suffice it to say, at this time he felt that taking general medical practice somehow into psychiatry would support the latter's association with psychology generally, and mainly from a psychotherapeutic perspective, as well as maintaining the body in the picture on its own terms, rather than in its limited view as the brain with the mind extending from it ... somehow. Although he would have to appreciate and manage severe mental disorders and understand the rationale and usage of medications for mental distress and illness, he felt this was a small price to pay in what seemed to be a unifying idea, if not as a career plan for him personally.

Although he didn't think that he would have much contact with severe mental health disorders after training, analysis did offer a forensic approach of a kind, so Kennan left the option open. Also, medication had a place not only for severe disorders, but in general mental distress as well. He saw its usage in this area to be temporary and supportive, rather than permanent, but believed his further knowledge in this area might prove valuable.

> The red-haired man did choose my ward. When he arrived, he demanded to see me: I had anticipated this and was prepared. Mick – he was of Irish descent after all – came into my office in a livid state. His features reminded me of an irate leprechaun. I had realised prior that I was dealing with an intelligent man, and I would need to continue to act cleverly and decisively. So, I took Mick into my confidence straight away.
>
> I had the benefit of some background. Mick had been in the unit before for another suicide attempt, which was also why he was in intensive care on this occasion. When he was admitted, it was not my rostered call day, but the registrar on call – also a trainee specialist – approached me to ask a favour: that I see Mick instead of him.
>
> The registrar explained that Mick had been under his care during his previous admission. He also explained that he found Mick more than he could manage and was not surprised he had repeated his suicide attempt. This explanation of vulnerability and admission of failure made the difference in my decision to see this new patient, when I had initially dismissed the registrar as a prick.
>
> So, unbeknownst to Mick, I had gone forewarned.
>
> My actions in intensive care were designed to

change the dynamic of the relationship between doctor and patient, which patently had not been successful on his previous admission. I explained this all to Mick at this first true meeting. As if a dial was turned down, Mick's anger quickly abated. I had his confidence and we had a rapport, though not without a little manipulation!

What stood behind the distress and suicide attempt was something a general practitioner might appreciate more than a trainee with no equivalent experience. Mick had been diagnosed with epilepsy and lost his driving license as a consequence. What I further determined was that Mick's epileptic fits – there had only been a few – were always associated with either marijuana or alcohol withdrawal states. There was no family history of epilepsy and he did not have a diagnostic pattern on testing of his brain.

Mick was devastated by the loss of license, and quite understandably in my opinion. During the hospital stay the rapport developed into a therapeutic relationship that focused mainly on safe drug usage, and Mick was eventually discharged. I assessed that he probably would need to remain symptom-free for two years to get his license back, but he seemed up to the challenge.

As the registrars went through a rotation process, I was not to follow up on Mick but would meet him at a later point in our respective travels. I had given Mick my phone number, as by this time I was aware that in a matter of months I would have left psychiatric training. Sometimes healing can take time, even a lifetime.

Kennan had told me the story as a kind of explanation about his attitude to psychiatry. Somehow the story became intermingled with the discussion about his career choice as well as where the various professions and their approaches fitted in the scheme of things. These lacked the kind of uniformity and apparent clarity present in medicine and other medical specialities. He now feels this is a commentary on the role of psychiatry as a medical speciality, as he gradually immersed himself in the anti-psychiatry school of belief and the positions that have emerged from this.

By the time Kennan saw Mick, he had already resigned from his post as a registrar and the psychiatric training process. He felt that gave him a license to deal with Mick in a way he might not have prior. He was a bit cavalier now, and this was also a reason why the registrar to whom Mick was originally allotted asked him to take on the case. Kennan found it interesting how such a cavalier approach is not generally acceptable until the chips are down, even though it would ultimately and ironically bring even he down.

At this point in the story, I could tell Kennan was on vulnerable ground, so I asked him how he had gotten to this point. I was well aware that there were other prior stories that he wanted to relate but, for some reason, he started with this one and proceeded backwards.

> My mentor, the psychiatric analyst I was working with, had died shortly before I met Mick. I found this out from another analytic trainee through a phone call, and it left me numb. I knew he had not been well, but his death came as a surprise and stopped me in my tracks. I also immediately realised it would cause a reassessment of my place as a psychiatric trainee and this would need to be rapid.

The mentorship with my analyst, I presumed, was known amongst the psychiatric community, hence my more 'dynamic' and psychotherapeutic proclivities were also well known. Although I had tried to disguise this fact and maintain a clear separation between my psychiatric and analytic training with my mentor, this was not always easy to do. Also, I am not naturally duplicitous – an irony in a speciality loaded with duplicity – so didn't try unduly to maintain any secrecy of my interests and intent.

Now, without this unseen support and protection, I was very exposed in many ways. I looked to alternatives, such as doing psychiatric training back in Britain, but an intense love interest that had me captivated effectively precluded this. Then I remembered a warning I had received from the registrar whose position I took over.

We were doing a patient handover, before I started my posting and were walking down the corridor to get a cup of tea, having completed the handover.

"By the way," she said, "don't fuck anyone on the psychiatric unit."

I was taken aback. She couldn't be referring to patients, as that was and is a very distinct no-no generally in medicine. She was referring to staff, and she clarified this by including administrative staff.

When she saw my shocked expression, she smiled. "It's all very well for you, I can't screw anyone else at all!"

She went on to explain that, although she was separated from her husband, this should make no difference. To whom? The blatant sexism in psychiatry notwithstanding, where did this edict come from? She then told me that there was a moral assessment that occurred at the completion of training. Apparently, there were a group of psychiatrists who, examination results notwithstanding, decided whether the trainee could enter the 'psychiatric club' – also referred to as the Royal Australian and New Zealand College of Psychiatrists – purely on moral grounds. This sort of policing is obviously very open to manipulation, at many levels. Need I say more?

What was my delayed response to this?

After I tendered my resignation, I duly slept with one of the occupational therapists, whom I knew one of the consultant psychiatrists fancied, but – theoretically – could not touch. There was definitely no turning back after that kind of somewhat ironic payback!

After my mentor's death, and prior to undertaking this course of action with the said therapist, I wanted to corroborate my stance within psychiatry before I made a decision. Mindful of my colleague's introductory warnings about the training, I made an appointment to see the Professor of Psychiatry.

At this meeting, I decided not to bring my analytic interests and the fact that I was now significantly advanced in training as an analyst. I suspected the professor was aware of at least my inclination and certainly my deceased mentor's patronage, but I did not want this to unduly influence the discussion. I wanted to focus purely on psychiatry and my place within it.

I explained my position along the lines of the difficulty my prior breadth of experience – being over three years of general practice – made to training, and then asked his advice. What surprised me was, the man immediately took this as a cue to recommend that

I leave. He covered this with all sorts of platitudes, which I accepted at the time, and he also gave me the impression that leaving was my own choice.

But many, many years later, I found out that my suspicions at the time were right: I was persona non-grata and without my mentor's support and protection I would be wasting my time going further with dual training. I met the professor in other circumstances and considered him to be seriously personality-disordered. But I am not a psychiatrist, so how can I make such a diagnosis?

In the several months of time I had remaining, I was now able to show my hand and explore a dynamic approach in the context of a psychiatric unit that was overwhelmingly organic in orientation. As well as, yes, bedding the therapist, although this was not a reaction; I genuinely found her attractive and she was now not prohibited territory. So, why not?

Our café discussion now took some light relief as we explored sexuality in psychiatry, and then extended this to medicine generally. A colleague had recently recounted an overseas study to Kennan, reporting that a slight majority of male psychiatrists had had at least one sexual encounter with a patient. He simply laughed.

"After my various experiences in both medicine and psychiatry, I think this may well be an underestimate!" He then went on to describe some of his knowledge and experience in this area that, even with my wide and varied experience, I found quite confronting.

We also wondered what the figure would be amongst female psychiatrists; whether the figure was reduced because of non-disclosure in spite of assurance regarding confidentiality, and what this figure would be amongst the medical profession generally. As one doctor friend, who was deregistered for a sexual relationship with a patient, was told by a colleague: "The only problem you have is that you got caught, unlike the rest of us!"

However, there was a level of authenticity to what Kennan had unravelled that was undeniable. The code of silence in the profession; the lack of sharing amongst colleagues about sexual issues, and the general policing of the issue that stuck us both as rigidly and duplicitously immoral, as well as being out of date, made this a difficult area to discuss with any sort of clarity.

And, as Kennan pointed out, since Freud at least, there has been a clear and open discussion about the relationship between sex, illness and disease, even though the impact of this discussion on medical practice per se is questionable. Therefore, sexuality would inevitably permeate any medical or therapeutic relationship.

Denial of this simple fact, and the outmoded belief that this can be dealt with by policing the professions is not only wrong, it is, in his opinion "just plain bad". It was also a denial of the role of the erotic in the medical relationship more generally, and specifically its potential as a channel of healing.

Kennan then went to a further story of a lawyer's wife whom he admitted to the ward early one morning, after her husband contacted him directly, imploring him to do so.

> Liz was an attractive young woman who was hand-wringing more than Lady Macbeth when I first saw her. Following a hunch, it didn't take long for me to ascertain that the depression she was experiencing was because of guilt regarding an extra-marital affair she was involved in.
>
> I admitted her to the ward consenting to my

consultant's plan of management, being electroconvulsive therapy – ECT – in addition to the already prescribed antidepressants. This was based on their combined success with a prior admission. This was with disquiet on my part when I read the notes of her previous admission, where the assessment was identical except that it described her as "sitting immobile in the chair"; no evidence of agitation, I noted, so something had changed in the meantime. There was no note of any marital infidelity, either, though given her husband's status, I did not know whether this was not known or not committed to record.

As the antidepressant drugs and ECT were patently not working, I decided that some counselling might be in order. So keen was Liz to absolve herself of the guilt that it required no great expertise on my part for her to make a confession, which I had suspected with her hand-wringing. She readily acquiesced to therapy and we were making good headway when my consultant decided it was time for discharge and, because she was privately insured, he referred her to a private psychiatrist for continuing therapeutic management as, in his opinion, he felt she needed a "father figure".

Of course, he had every justification in the book for this, but I was quietly annoyed and concerned. The therapy I was conducting was progressing well. It also contained what is known in the trade as 'transference', when the patient transfers unresolved emotional feelings onto the therapist. Inevitably, and with her prior history and marital dissatisfaction, I became the object of this attention. I was both aware of this and quite capable of working with it; in fact, I saw such an approach as essential to her healing process. Then my fucking consultant interfered.

Many weeks later, I was to readmit her after a serious suicide attempt, whilst she was still in therapy with the private psychiatrist. I took a more pragmatic approach on this occasion, because anything else would have been frankly dangerous. When she was again discharged, I gave her instructions about how I could be directly contacted on the unit, if ever she needed. Her husband seemed to have such a privilege, after all.

One phone call some months later was to reassure me. Then, some years later, I was to meet her in an educational workshop. She was happy, vital and ... single. Did we consummate her previous attraction? No, because in my mind that had never been the nature of the relationship, and not simply because she was my patient. And she had come to realise this too. The reconnection was pleasing and intimate, and we were to go our own ways. Some weeks later I received a book from her. It was a delightfully notated signed book of poetry by a poet we both admired.

"Well, that's dealt with sex," said Kennan, "or at least as far as we can take it for now."

His wink unnerved me a little, but he went on: "So I think we should get to death!" Not only was he a rebel, a maverick, he had a devilish sense of humour. In the early days of our meetings, I reflected that I would have taken that remark quite differently.

It wasn't until we next met that Kennan told his story about death or, more specifically, suicide. In contrast to the mood in which he had finished our last conversation, he was more sombre. It wasn't too long before I realised why: he had a big tale to tell, and full of ramifications beyond the psychiatric.

He told me it had also occurred prior to the accounts above, so probably had a defining effect on the way Kennan conducted himself subsequently, as well as his decision to leave psychiatry. It may also have been a further influence on his professor's attitude when reinforced by a chance piece of information he was to hear many months later.

> I was on call, but after hours this was commonly a quiet affair. The casualty staff knew that the evening and night presentations were often more psychosocial than psychiatric, and so the residents there usually took an interim measure, such as a sedative and a bed for the anxious patient. Then the on-call registrar would start early the next day and assess the overnight haul. Were we "fishers of men"? I pondered.
>
> I had just finished a hard game of squash and was settling down to an evening meal cooked by my lover, when I received a call from casualty. There was a patient there who would need to be admitted. The patient had been sent from a private psychiatric hospital by a psychiatrist in private practice. I was enraged – at this ungodly hour? Why hadn't the psychiatrist at least given me prior warning, or the decency of an earlier phone call?
>
> I didn't change and went to casualty in my sports gear, leaving dinner – and the possible desserts – in the oven. There was a brief note from the psychiatrist; something about the patient being suicidal, and that he would give more details the next day. This never eventuated. The man had been under the psychiatrist's care for some months.
>
> This was all starting to smell. The man was depressed and suicidal, yes, but I gained little else from the initial interview, except that he was an adopted

child with no family history available. His partner was close to giving birth to their own first child, and she had a young son at home from a previous relationship.

One thing did surprise me. At the end of the interview, I asked Aaron how he had experienced me. Arrogant, was Aaron's reply. I was taken aback. Angry maybe, although I'd done my best to discharge this before the interview, but arrogant in sports gear and a simple desire to facilitate the process expediently? Again, what this may have meant only came to light later.

Over the next few days, Aaron was observed. Surprisingly, my own consultant had taken no interest in the case, even though he was from private sources and hence a potential income avenue for him; this was something he forewent rarely. And, as little was drawn from the staff on the ward about Aaron's attitude and behaviour, I approached him and arranged that we meet and discuss his situation and management further in the forthcoming days. He was enthusiastic about this.

After the intervening weekend, I came into the ward on Monday morning to find an agitated relative of Aaron's wanting to see me. I asked him to sit and wait whilst I dealt with the transfer of a patient, who had become manic and would be uncontrollable on an open ward such as mine. The relative sat quietly through this interruption, but the tension was palpable.

Then he simply told me that he had found Aaron, and asked me to accompany him. I had not even known Aaron was absent. But an older experienced English male psychiatric nurse knew, picked up on what was happening, and accompanied the two of us.

We made our way across the road to the neighbouring Kings Park where Aaron was hanging by the neck from a tree. He was dead. His feet were on the ground, but he had deep cuts in his forearms. He probably inflicted these and passed out prior to asphyxiating. The relative abruptly turned and left.

What a mess. The next few days I was numb.

Then I heard news that a second male patient recently discharged from the unit, who was under my consultant's care as he was a doctor's son, had also hung himself. Mark had gone to a hardware store, bought some rope on his father's account, and then committed the act. As with Aaron, there was no explanatory note. I barely knew Mark, but he had a reputation on the ward as being a troublemaker.

After my consultant had brought myself and any involved others together, he asked us to go through Mark's clinical notes and correct anything that may have been inaccurate or incorrect. I was troubled by this, in spite of all the consultant's reasoning; he was obviously troubled too. Later, I did my own investigation, because the smell now became a stink.

Mark had shared a double room with Aaron. It was known that the former talked a lot about how he was going to kill himself, but it was widely believed – prior to Aaron's death – that he was attention-seeking and being manipulative. The reasons behind this were unknown to me, as I wasn't managing Mark's case, although it was obvious that Aaron was and would have been the recipient of and receptive to this talk.

I now put two and two together and came up with a plausible pattern of events. Aaron was tipped over the edge by all this, and then, maybe racked with guilt now, Mark committed a similar act. He was discharged only a day or so after Aaron's death. Neither myself nor my consultant, knew they roomed together. The pall over the unit was palpable. But what was most surprising, some weeks later when I presented the situation at a case conference on the unit, the medical staff were only interested in diagnoses and not the whole psychosocial background.

The psychiatric nurse, who had accompanied me to Aaron's body, took me to one side and said: "Watch where the next suicide occurs."

I asked him what he meant, but he implied that, once I left the unit, I would find out that the problem was on the unit itself, and not to see it as my own. The inference toward the consultant was clear.

But I did take it personally. A couple of days after Aaron's death I received a belated call from Aaron's referring private psychiatrist.

"How's that young man I sent you last week?"

"He hanged himself over the weekend."

"Oh dear, oh dear. I knew he would do that. That's why I sent him to you."

I put ... slammed ... the phone down. *You arrogant psychopathic bastard ... Arsehole; fucking, fucking arsehole!*

My thinking about the man was hardly polite. Many months later I had a casual conversation with another consultant, Greg, about a different patient:

"This case is like the one that was sent to you, remember, Kennan? The guy who killed himself. It was well-known around town that he was going to do that. It is why he was sent to a public hospital."

And I had drawn the short straw. Now I knew another strand in my professor's attitude toward me.

Was the arrogance about me that Aaron remarked upon the referring psychiatrist's or his own?

Kennan would like to think the former, but maybe a bit of both. Over time, the whole incident helped define for him what his ultimate decision would be. He would leave psychiatry, continue with his analytic training, and start a private practice as a psychotherapist. In the last weeks of his registrar post, he started the translation with a little bit of private psychotherapeutic practice on the side, which he could then build on when he left.

Yet the whole incident troubled Kennan then, and it continues to do so. He has maintained an interested perspective of psychiatry generally, but a more distant and wary one about psychiatric practice in his home city of Perth, particularly since he left. At that time, he felt he had enough diagnostic ability and pharmaceutical knowledge in the area to take into private psychotherapeutic practice, but he decided not to use hospitals. So, for that and other reasons, he maintained some contact with the one or two private psychiatrists he liked and could trust.

Aaron's death remains a mystery at one level. Kennan felt it was bound up with being an adoptive child from unknown biological parents, and who was shortly to have his own child. If so, there were some deep reasons involved that would only become clearer to him as time progressed. Yet ultimately the choice for Aaron to kill himself remains a sad one, and a huge lesson for him.

Unlike the previous chapter, describing Kennan's journey through his years in general practice that I was able to understand and resonate with, the whole account of this chapter left me confused and troubled. In some ways, I saw sides to his character that reminded me of some of my earlier concerns. But here they were in a moral and ethical context that made me see them – and him – in a quite different light.

Maybe that was what troubled me: the moral and ethical

issues raised here were more immediate and personal. I am left deeply troubled about psychiatry; but I have been so for many years, so Kennan demonstrates here that this may be more than a simply local effect, medically, socially, and politically, but indicates a far more concerning trend about psychiatry in – at least – the western world.

Now I felt I was naming the confusion: it is not about psychiatry or even medicine. It is about the social, legal, political, and ethical frameworks within which psychiatry is embedded. If my reasoning is correct, it paints a very bleak, and even a sick, picture. I can see now why Kennan left. But I am sure the traces of this chapter will weave their way down the ongoing account.

Six

Kennan had made a clear decision. He had come to the inexorable conclusion that an organic or biomechanically-based psychiatry was not for him. He actually wondered whether it was for anyone, doctor or patient, but this was only a nascent thought at that time. Instead, he considered the more dynamic and psychotherapeutic branch of psychiatry was what interested him; it talked to him. But to achieve this, he would either have to go through the five-year psychiatric training programme and qualify as a specialist to then branch out, or go overseas and train in psychiatry in an institution that was more conducive to the dynamic branch.

The alternative was to move away from psychiatry completely, and then explore the dynamic branch outside of institutional medicine by pursuing training as an analyst, whilst remaining under the broader general medical practitioner umbrella with a self-restricted practice, as well as keeping the physical body in the overall picture; something he believed psychiatry only paid limited and token homage to.

Kennan followed his heart and took the latter option. A year as a registrar in psychiatry had given him sufficient diagnostic skills, as well as enough understanding of the medications used in the psychiatric realms. This would prove useful; he was the only medically trained person in his group of analysts in the discipline of Carl Jung in Western Australia at the time. Called Analytical Psychology by Jung, to distinguish it from Freud's Psychoanalysis, he was about halfway through his analytic training when he left psychiatry. Now, with his exclusive focus here and a private medical practice that was entirely psychotherapeutic in orientation, he felt settled.

The pressure was also markedly reduced. Kennan worked from home, seeing up to forty clients a week (he preferred and still prefers the term 'client' to 'patient' in this area) and his own training was based around himself being further analysed with a training analyst. He now had no formal medical associations at the practitioner level. The only medically and psychiatrically trained analysts were elsewhere in Australia. He was also reliant on the local network that existed around Jung's work for many referrals. Though none of this network was medically trained, there were a couple of clinical psychologists in the group.

Kennan estimated that, by the time he started private psychotherapeutic practice, he had been in analysis himself for over 150 one-hour sessions with three analysts. He was currently working with a woman-training analyst with whom he would complete the further minimum 150 hours necessary. In addition, he would be supervised with case material of his own for up to 100 hours. His reading and research followed his own analysis and what emerged from this, he was also expected to complete a thesis of substance when he submitted himself for qualification. But this would all take a further three years, so his private practice and his personal life were the main focuses in the meantime.

From my point of view, I had plenty of queries: "Did you feel socially isolated from medicine?" I asked.

By this stage of our relationship, I found that the flow between us had changed from one of an interchange of views and perspectives to my asking questions and getting into more of a dialogue from that point on. So, with respect to this account, I decided to change the format and use quotation marks, so that this dialogue could be better followed. Henceforth, I would change between these formats as the flow of conversation demanded, usually chapter by chapter.

Kennan's response was immediate. "Not at all. The year in psychiatry was fairly bruising. I felt I had been burnt, then burned my bridges to keep ahead of the fire."

I found his choice of metaphors to be multi-layered.

"I was to catch up with my psychiatry professor on two further occasions over the years. This confirmed my decision. I found the man at least duplicitous, or there was something about me that affected him. I have no doubt now that I was manipulated out of the psychiatric training programme after these subsequent meetings, being some kind of perceived threat.

"I recall our professor giving the registrars a lecture on one occasion, when he came out with some interesting evidence about schizophrenia. It was about the birth dates of schizophrenics having an annual numerical peak that varied in the yearly calendar over a significant time period of up to 100 years. He then added that he had to give this information because it was documented, even though it was incompatible with the existing – in fact any – scientific model.

"At tea, I sat with him and commented that the data was interesting, as it could be considered astrological and to follow the progression of the equinoxes. From a rationalistic perspective, I was putting the data in the quasi-mystical category.

"I thought you might say something like that." This was all I got as a reply, apart from a steely gaze.

"I had effectively left hospital practice and specialist training options; decided that general practice was not for me; realised psychiatry as I had experienced it was dysfunctional, so now my options came down to moving on with Jung and see where that path may take me. I remained medically registered, and my clients were able to gain healthcare rebates because they were experiencing psychological distress, but my contact with medicine in an active professional way was marginal.

"By contrast, Jung opened up so many avenues, personally and professionally. I was also living very much in the moment. I was absorbed in my own personal analysis and where that was leading me, both psychologically and spiritually, such that medicine seemed a long way away. And I found Jung exciting. I was not so enamoured with Jungians though … but we'll get to that I suspect."

"You felt more at peace professionally?" I queried, somewhat rhetorically.

"In general, yes. I was practising from home and did my own appointment bookings and book-keeping. I didn't require anything or anyone else. This setting was comfortable for clients as well as myself, and taught me a lot about the place of settings in healing – that is, where we conduct treatments.

"My clientele came mainly by word of mouth, although most were aware I had a Jungian inclination. My analytic colleagues sent some people for assessment from a psychiatric perspective, or to ascertain whether medication was indicated or necessary. Some clients were already on medication and I gained a reputation fairly rapidly for getting people off psychiatric drugs. Most times they weren't indicated, or the person had been misdiagnosed, and also psychotherapy lessens the need for drugs.

"This was not just psychiatric drugs. Remember Mick? Well, he had another seizure and had been put on anti-epileptic drugs since he left my care. He was also now not allowed to drive for a further two years, as I recall. Mick then got in contact with me and we started a therapy process that was to last three years. In that time, he got off his drugs and remained symptom-free to the point that he regained his license without medication.

"As an aside, Mick is an example of something all good psychotherapists know; that therapy can heal many cases of epilepsy because of its strong association with psychological stress and its management. I also know Mick remained well for over a decade after I stopped seeing him. How do I know this? Because he met someone I knew independently, married her, and settled down to family life with a newborn."

We had a break and I renewed the coffee order before proceeding.

"Three years is a long time for psychotherapy, isn't it?"

"Yes, or it seems to be. But Mick is an example of the potential benefits, notwithstanding that his neurologist had no knowledge of the benefits of psychotherapy. The fact that a medical specialist treating brain disorders does not have this sort of information at hand shows the relative isolation most medical specialties – including psychiatry – exist and operate within. Many psychotherapeutic managements simply take that long. At this stage in my career, the longer form was less marginalised than it is now, where the focus has progressively moved to quick results and the belief that 'cognitive' and 'behavioural' changes are all that is required.

"This is patently not the case and the evidence is beginning to show it. Long-term psychotherapy is getting a belated re-evaluation. It has its place, but the assessment of suitability is important. And this depends on the individual, not the condition. I have always been a strong advocate of longer-term psychotherapy, and with all the vicissitudes that medicine and psychology have undergone in my journey, this has remained a constant for me. I think you will find that many priests, who directly or indirectly conduct long-term psychotherapy, would agree."

"What makes you so adamant about long-term psychotherapy; because it can start to get costly, and why do you not select the condition or problem as the criterion for choice of therapy?" I was starting to feel we were getting into territory that needed further clarification.

"I think you've rolled at least two questions into one there! I'll go with the first part, as that extends from what I was saying previously.

"My own therapy was long-term; eventually well over 300 hours, and over a six-year period. I think the more personal therapy lasted until I made the decision to move to psychiatry, so say 100 or so hours. The remaining hours were more explorative in the psychospiritual sense. Usually, a therapy session is an hour a week. At today's rates, the rebate means that the therapy costs about $10,000.00. This sounds a lot, but compare it to the cost of hospital beds, psychiatric rates of charging (often $300 or more an hour), medication costs, allied care (psychologists and social workers) then this figure pales into relative insignificance.

"I still do not know of any comparative studies on what I have outlined. And, in the many years I was in full-time psychotherapy practice, I reckon I conducted 15,000 hours of therapy. The total is now at least 25,000 hours and my experience remains relatively isolated professionally, although this is not unusual with practitioners like myself. By any standards, this is an appreciable experiential base for informed input.

"More than this is my own anecdotal evidence. I have seen many Micks and for a plethora of conditions, both physical and psychological, although I now do not differentiate the two. I have often seen the medical and psychiatric failures – maybe one reason nobody asks me too often – the cases that have been parked on drugs and are in the 'too hard' basket. I have seen the rewards of my approach, by comparison. Sure, I have also seen and experienced the failures, but each one makes me ask questions of myself first, rather than of the client. This is what personal therapy taught me, and is something that trainee psychiatrists do not routinely undergo.

"Let me finish with an example. When I was in general practice before moving to psychiatry, I saw a businessman with an addiction to the sedative valium. He had been given it for work-related stress. When I first saw Dave, I listened to his story and came to the conclusion that he was intensely fixated on his mother. Then valium made sense, breast milk to soothe him when distressed, I reasoned.

"But I also listened to Dave's dreams, which talked about the dysfunctional relationship with his father. I was in a quandary; I wanted to deal with his obvious 'mother complex', but his dreams pointed elsewhere. I was a bit miffed, but we dealt with his father and within four weeks he was drug-free. And I was amazed, as I felt that his relationship with his mother was the root of his addictive problem.

"Then I forgot about him, until a couple of years later when I was now in private practice. He felt like he wanted to start taking the sedatives again, but also thought to approach me first. We agreed to meet and this time his mother came into the therapeutic picture, big time! So, I was right in my diagnosis, but wrong in my timing. I needed a good dose of patience. We continued work for several months and I knew some years down the track that he was still free of medication, as well as being in better and changed life circumstances; the latter is an inevitable consequence of good therapy, I might add."

There were questions that even this response raised. What were the criteria for choosing long-term psychotherapy? What were the reasons that mainstream had tended to neglect it? Was it because mainstream didn't see it to be effective, or of value, or for other reasons? As I considered these questions, I had the feeling that Kennan would probably cover them in the course of this account, although I also had the sense that some were not answerable in the way I had framed them; particularly the third question I posed — to myself — here. I allowed him to simply proceed with the earlier question.

"There is an enigmatic thing in the core of all this, called consciousness. In the past, although the idea lingers on, there was seen to be a separation between consciousness and unconsciousness. Even though I was trained in a tradition that, coming in the wake of Freud, still used this distinction, I have always found it problematic. I have progressively avoided using the word 'unconscious' in the psychological sphere, but I need to explain why.

"When I trained, consciousness was fairly synonymous with our day-to-day reality, that some may even term 'self or ego-consciousness'. But if I have problems with the word 'unconscious', then I have even more problem with 'ego'! I think — now — we have a consciousness that is oriented in daily reality and that is defined by time, space, and various other familiar parameters. But I think this limited consciousness, or 'self', like the tip of an iceberg, rests on top of a greater consciousness, which we experience in dreams, mystical states, or other so-called altered states of consciousness, including with the use of drugs, also with intuition, synchronicity or 'serendipity'. In fact, the iceberg image is probably wrong, because this larger view of consciousness is that it is ultimately without limit. I'm sure others can draw a better model from quantum physics though, as it is one I have been progressively drawn to.

"Cognitive and other similar more mechanical and scientific therapies are aimed at expanding and bolstering that daily consciousness only. And, with various distortions and traumas in our early development, this could be a good place to start and is sufficient for a lot of people. But there are some, a minority I admit, who have what is called 'insight'. They know there is more to life than daily reality and for a variety of intersecting reasons, either innately, or in their development; but they do know this. And you can't negate this insight, so cognitive approaches won't work beyond a point, if at all, with this grouping. They need approaches that work on the relationship between the consciousness of daily reality and that of the greater reality – in which the daily one exists, by the way!

"Okay, enough philosophy and mysticism; what does this mean practically? It means that it is not the problem that determines the correct therapy, but the consciousness, awareness or insight of the individual, or all three perhaps. What I do when I assess someone for psychotherapy is gauge this first. If it is not there, I refer on to a cognitive psychologist or someone else appropriate. If it is, then the degree and strength of it can be guessed at, although I am always surprised! But, if there, it's then enough to start and just get cracking with therapy.

"How do you assess insight and its degree? Well, does the client dream? If so, what is the quality and their interest in them? Are they creative? Do they keep a diary or journal? Do they have a strong intuition, experience coincidences, and respond to unusual events? Are they considered a bit odd, eccentric, or even mad by those around them – particularly family? But importantly, it depends on the insight of the therapist. Don't forget that a therapist in this mould has been through an extensive period of therapy him or herself and this involves forging the relationship between these two intersecting realities – if that's an understandable way of terming it. So, they would recognise this potential more readily in another."

"You haven't talked about how the 'condition or problem', as I referred to it, affects or dictates the mode of therapy," I interjected. After a refill of coffee, Kennan surprised me with how he started his response.

"One of the reasons I left psychiatry was because I realised that psychiatrists, in general, had lost contact with the body.

They had taken the mind and body duality to an extreme and set themselves up as specialist of the mind, usually exclusively, but by using models of the body as applied to the mind, and not the models of the mind on its own terms. Whilst even the physical medical specialities are starting to have trouble with this mechanical viewpoint of the body, imagine what it is like for a speciality like psychiatry that cannot even be conceived like this in the first place!

"Now there are several problems with this, foremost of which is separating the mind and body in the first place. The older and more experienced I get, the less I see it that way and can't separate them. But, as indicated just now, the major problem is that psychiatry sees problems in the way we look at problems of the body. And this is scientifically, mechanically, and standing firmly outside of the problem emotionally. This last factor is emerging of great importance in other disciplines; the role of subjectivity is being reassessed and included. I hope in the near future medicine will start to embrace these developments.

"Because long-term psychotherapy, or the discipline of depth psychology that it is considered to be an expression of, has known this about emotion for a long time. The early psychoanalysts saw it in terms of something called 'transference' and based on a principle called 'projection'. I could go a lot further here, but it gets away from the point, which is that this process has become more fluid and subtle. I now see that the therapist and client exist together in some sort of fundamental unity that maybe the therapist understands and can navigate a bit better.

"I think I'm getting to your question slowly, Ian, but these other points keep arising first. So, I guess they might be significant. Or I'm just worried I may not get to discuss them, or that you might not ask a relevant question!"

I think I did warn the reader earlier about how Kennan's mind works ...

Kennan has some interesting views about psychiatry, but foremost amongst these is the way mental distress is perceived, understood, and managed.

"The one thing about your own therapy is that you get to see your own problems in a stark way, where you can't easily wriggle out of them or blame anyone else, because a good therapist won't let you. These problems are usually ones that create discomfort for us, and we experience them emotionally in either mind or body, or actually both. Emotion is a tell-tale sign of something below the surface of your own mind that is creating disturbance and wanting to be heard.

"If it creates too much disturbance, we may want it to go away, so we avoid it, take medication or pursue addictive pathways. But it has its say anyway and, if we don't listen, it may manifest in the body. Now this is where insight comes in. Painful though it may be, we have to own the discomfort or distress and figure out what it is 'telling' us: because it is telling us something. The mind is exquisitely crafted; it doesn't create unrest for no reason, even if it may disturb our daily equilibrium and personal agendas.

"Mental distress is not a disease; it is really 'mental stress'. It may lead to disordered behaviour and problems like addiction, but there is no such thing as a mental disease. All mental disturbance is just that: Disturbance. We have yet to find a single objective fact in our scientific endeavours that defines any mental state as a disease in the definitive sense. And we won't. I'm aware such a comment is against the current trend and also brings in such issues as religion and morality. But we will have to get used to opening up our mindsets, as the medical paradigm undergoes essential changes, even a transformation.

"What I found, all those years ago, was that it didn't matter what it was that the client had as a distress. They may present themselves with anxiety, obsessive-compulsive disorder, depression or an addiction. Usually, and not helped by either the profession or the media, they see this as 'other' than themselves. An anxiety 'they have', as if it is a foreign invader, similar to a virus.

"One of the problems here is we see the mind and brain as being the same. They are not. The brain is an organ in the body, like the liver or kidneys. The mind is not tangible in the same way. That the mind and brain have a relationship there can be no doubt. But now when we are in an era that sees that we have brain-like connections in the gut and heart, we should start to revision the brain and mind, as most other non-medical disciplines have done.

"One way to start this unravelling process is to appreciate that the mind is more than our cognitive and sensate abilities, and that we need to understand ourselves emotionally, intellectually, and even spiritually. These functions cannot be easily restricted to the brain, which is probably one reason that the scientific community excludes them. It sees anxiety to be a disorder of brain chemistry, maybe genetically driven, but rectifiable with an appropriate chemical adjustment.

"The trouble is that these adjustments don't work well, except symptomatically sometimes and temporarily for the short-term; although for whose benefit is a question in itself. In fact, over the longer term, they create all sorts of problems like addiction, permanent brain side-effects, social isolation, and dysfunction generally. They gloss over the problems; they don't fix them … because they can't by definition.

"This is where therapy of some sort comes in. It deals with the psychological, social, family, occupational, and even spiritual aspects of a person's existence. And we all have all of them, and they all impact on our health, most detectable mentally. But what therapy? Is it temporary, superficial, requiring a cognitive approach only? Or is it deep, requiring the attendance of a priest? Is the modern psychotherapist part both, depending on his or her disposition and that of the client?

"I have simply found that long-term psychotherapy worked irrespective of the so-called 'condition'. Because it depends for its success on other factors such as insight, responsibility, and the client making an effort and taking some risks. Risks are interesting because it is something both client and therapist engage in, and this brings up all sorts of undercurrents that may become part of the engagement, the relationship. When this gets to shadowy material like anger and sexuality, the ride can be bumpy.

"Also, a focus on the presenting problem exclusively may miss the point, as it might simply represent something deeper and other, which may need the sort of decoding a good therapy can undertake. Such decoding demands an appreciation of a layered mentality, with the appreciation of metaphor and symbolism, euphemism and humour. I have also found that the longer the therapy the more permanent the changes and hence the healing. But it is not an easy path; it is no surprise we collectively search and opt for simpler methods, the trouble being that they don't work long term."

Kennan then went on to say that he now, more than ever, appreciated why he couldn't become a psychiatrist. "Because psychiatry generally ignores the body," he stated. "I never lost those years in medicine and general practice where I started to see psychological and social problems emerge from the physical. So, I reasoned it was a two-way process: unravel the physical to get to the psychological, and beyond, as well as vice versa."

In this, he was enunciating a truth that many have and had come to. It is just that he saw long-term psychotherapy as inclusive of the body in a way most others didn't. His career in general medicine had given him that advantage or benefit, it seemed to me.

What I wasn't clear about in this wide-ranging discussion was how much Kennan's thoughts were an expression of how he felt at the time – this being now well over thirty years ago – and his current thinking. He said he had wondered this too and had come to the conclusion that they were his present thoughts, but born of the embryo that is within his account. He likened it to looking at a photograph of himself at that time. He is both surprised at how he looked then, but also sees a connection with the present. But although he obviously cannot truly put himself back to that time, he explained it in this way:

"When I form an image of that time and recall any memories, I have the feeling that I actually 'go back' into them and 'see' the events as I recall them, yet with another aspect of myself watching from the present, at the same time. So, when I recall these memories, they feel alive and I find myself using the language, impressions and thoughts that were there then. Because whenever I have had the opportunity to undertake this process before meeting you, I have been surprised at the words and terms I use. They seem archaic to the 'me' in the present, and I have an urge to correct or update them, which I resist. I believe they are as faithful to the time as they can be, for myself anyway."

Kennan even broadened this scope to the problems his clients brought to him. He says that they heal, but don't cure. And by cure he means going back to a time before the malaise or problem occurred. He maintains that is impossible and that all illness changes us. He even sees that as one of its functions. So, the memories and their recall, even if traumatic, which they inevitably are in this sphere, can heal us; if we can but reconcile them in the present to move forward. He sees this as transformative, in contrast to being confined and defined by our wounds and the memories of them. At this point I raised my eyebrow I suspect, because he smiled, told me not to worry, that we'd come back to this point.

I was now beginning to trust the man, because he did come back to these points when necessary and weave them into the account. It is part of his style, his disposition, something in the deep trust he has in narrative. I started to see him in an old term: Wordsmith. There was even something poetic about his account. But one significant thing that was emerging clearly was that his view of time and its role in illness and disease was not the same as our conventional notions. To this we would return, I had no doubt.

To complete this session together I asked Kennan where he felt he was now placed in his account.

"Ah," he responded, "I was just wondering that myself! I think I have jumped a few years, maybe five. I have a lot of stories from those days as an analyst."

Kennan qualified as an analyst three years after he left psychiatry. He had a maturing analytic orientation that continued to develop from his psychotherapeutic practice, which continued unabated, but with the added qualification. This period was to continue for three further years before life directed him elsewhere.

It is not that there were no stories, he reassured me, but they did not seem – now – to have the significance they might have had at the time. There was an evenness about his work then. It was stable and predictable, and people liked that, and he tried to make himself like it as well, although there were some rumblings in the basement that he could detect. There were also wider educational and teaching functions he was now involved in, including lectures, workshops and conferences.

In fact, the only stories that sprung to his mind, Kennan told me, were ones that involved colleagues with vested interests, distortions in analytic training, and the occasional interference from the psychiatric world. These carried many of the dynamics and implications that he felt he had covered in his time in psychiatry, somewhat disconcertingly, and maybe also foretold that his time in this field itself may be limited.

Kennan reflected deeply. Then he told me that there was maybe only one story within practice itself that was now relevant to share publicly. The rest could be the subject of a personal analytic journal, but not the sort that was an integral part of this account.

> I had been seeing Jane for several months. She was very attractive, even beautiful, and single. She had the habit of negating men with derision, but after a couple of glasses of wine and when ovulating, she was in danger. I advised her about contraception, but at the wrong time of her cycle; she was dismissive claiming she would never need them because she did not intend sleeping with a man "ever again".
>
> And so, we continued. We dealt with her work and her creativity, and settled into the sort of comfort an analytic relationship can, which is always dangerous. She was sitting on a powder keg and I didn't have any idea when it would blow. I thought it was pregnancy that was the danger. I was wrong. One day she came at dusk and we settled into the analytic rhythm.
>
> "I had a dream. It was about a huge spider," she said. Her mother, I thought, about time! Then silence.
>
> It was as if we were both hypnotised when she exclaimed through a shocked and ashen expression: "Get it out!" pointing past me to the corner of the room. And then I looked to the corner and could see the

spider. It was gigantic. We were both deeply shocked as the image faded.

Jane became very angry with me subsequent to this experience. It built up in one session when she stormed out, without a word. I intuitively knew she would try and kill herself. The next thing I knew I was walking to the phone. I was going to ring a psychiatric consultant mentor I had kept contact with and tell him; mainly to cover myself legally, but also because I liked his input … and he mine. But I couldn't pick up the phone. In a psychic way, I knew if I did I would be betraying Jane.

She arrived on schedule the next week, and I was – pleasantly – surprised. She told me she had been so angry with me and didn't know why. She left our session and drove to a local beach. It was getting dark and very stormy. She took off all her clothes and walked into the ocean, determined to get beyond the waves and drown. She was so angry; angry with me. But the waves wouldn't let her get that far, she was repeatedly thrown back. Resigned, she went home and drank herself to sleep instead.

Jane wasn't angry as she told me this; she even smiled. Something had broken and all would be well. And for Jane, it would be so, as I found with an overseas call from her some years later.

Kennan looked into the distance.

"Now I know why I told you this story, Ian; it was a sign of what was to come."

Seven

Ann's death was surprisingly the next topic for discussion. Surprising because we now jumped several years in the overall account, and also because Kennan chose it with a kind of announcement when we met. He had obviously thought about this since our previous meeting a week before, probably provoked by the account about Jane.

As the story of their relationship and her death was to prove predictably erratic from any sort of ordered perspective, I feel it pertinent to put a time frame in place before starting. This was because I was becoming accustomed to the mazes that Kennan would wander into, although I trusted this would be more like a labyrinth and we would discover something important in it.

Kennan met Ann just over three years before her death. This was shortly after the point that we finished at in the previous meeting's discussion. As she was only ill for the latter three months of her life, and died seven months after the diagnosis, there is a period of a little over three years that he has jumped, which encompassed the entirety of their relationship. I suspect he will return to them, but he obviously sees fit to preface this period with her illness and death, rather than taking my preferred linear approach. Such is Kennan.

The diagnosis was a little under a week after the uneventful birth of their daughter, Asha. The actual circumstances around the birth were eventful enough, though. Ann and Kennan were having the birth at home, as they had with their son, Chaz, nearly two years previously. The same midwife was to provide assistance, there was another mutual friend as support, and all the necessary preparations were completed several days before.

Then on the day Asha was due, Kennan was awoken to the sound of furious sweeping. It was pouring with rain and he found Ann at the rear of the house trying to deal with a torrent of water that was cascading down the hill into the house. But it was a literal torrent and obviously well beyond Ann's efforts. He remembered she was short-sighted and she was surprised when he pointed out that her efforts were in vain. So instead, he went to the front of the house to inspect further.

Down the hill at the front, the brook had burst its banks and with it, the bridge over it had been washed away. This was their only vehicle connection to the outside world. Under the bridge, the water pipe was broken and upstream the electricity conduit was vulnerable. Kennan just sincerely hoped Ann would not go into labour that day.

But she did that night. It was a few minutes after Kennan went to bed exhausted after a steak and a surfeit of red wine. He had spent the day downstream locating the beams from the bridge, hauling them back and constructing a passage of sorts, should it be needed. The water had begun to subside and he was able to recreate a passable bridge. He also hauled some fresh water up in containers and made sure they had plenty of candles, should the power fail.

Asha's birth was the least eventful event of the day or, more correctly, the early hours of the next day. The labour was only four hours; Ann gathered Asha up and took her to bed with her from the delivery area in front of the fire. The midwife, our support lady, and Kennan went to their respective beds and slept. They all needed it; except Ann, whose focus was on the new arrival.

These events, a bare story in embryo but never to become fully fleshed, were superseded by what was to follow. As Ann began breastfeeding, she experienced difficulty in encouraging

Asha to suckle from one breast, as the nipple was not as prominent as on the other. This had not been the case with Chaz; she then told Kennan that her nipple had become like this for the latter weeks of the pregnancy, as her breasts started to prepare for feeding the newborn. Kennan became concerned over the ensuing day or so when the nipple remained 'inverted' in spite of Asha's attention, so Ann's obstetrician was contacted.

Although Ann had decided on a homebirth, she had an obstetrician oversee the pregnancy and any problems that might emerge. He, sight unseen, referred Ann immediately to a surgeon. Alarm bells started going off everywhere, although Kennan could feel nothing abnormal in Ann's breast. Nor could the surgeon, although he immediately referred her for an immediate needle biopsy.

I will pass the account over to Kennan now.

> Ann's breathing was very laboured. The small bedroom smelled of the fungating cancer that had broken through the skin and by now had entirely replaced the breast. How did it get to this?
>
> I recalled the days that followed the biopsy. I was on the train returning to our hillside home from Avalon House, the holistic health centre where I worked in West Perth, the professional area of the central business district of the city. The biopsy had been that day; it was possible the results could be negative, but what if they were not? I had thought this earlier, and I hoped against hope that they would be, but deep in my being the concern was ferocious. I imagined: Let's use this time of the 'unknown' to wrestle with the consequences of either option then, if the results are negative, we don't lose sight of something that may be important.

I didn't know it then, but I had stepped into a world better described by the 'indeterminacy' of quantum physics – Schrödinger's cat was both alive and dead, it would seem.

The surgeon rang at work two days later and gave me the news that all three biopsies were positive for aggressive breast cancer. It was 10.30 a.m. and I knew Ann was going to ring him at 11.00. Our home was over thirty minutes away, so I could not be there at home in time to tell her before she rang the surgeon. I bit the bullet, rang and told her the results; she was quiet and emotionally distant. I put the phone down, collapsed and cried before my secretary aroused me to begin the trek home.

There was a friend of Ann's there, who had supported Asha's birth, and she was crying. Ann was impassive, and distant as if she wasn't there at all. At that time, I knew she was going to die, and my first thought was 'please don't make it long and protracted'; don't act for the benefit of others, as we had both seen many with cancer do. But, in this respect, Ann was not typical, she was not consciously a victim. However, events were to prove that ultimately the illness was about being just that, although not in a way that was obvious to either of us at the time.

The obstetrician metaphorically washed his hands. "I thought you were checking the breasts," he said on a phone call, passing responsibility over to me. The dickhead! But that thought was brief, I simply consigned it – and him – to the past, as there were more important things to face. Ann had decided not to have surgery. The surgeon agreed he could manage her even if she didn't, but his body language said quite the opposite to me when we met. Later, I called on another surgeon, a friend I had met in my Colchester days in England, who agreed to act as a support.

The medicine was in place should it be needed, although we both knew it wouldn't be. Ann had made that clear and I was relieved; I knew modern western medicine had little to offer, and my more recent research only served to confirm this. Also, my surgeon friend backed these views – although privately and off the record, of course.

A couple of days after the biopsy diagnosis I examined Ann's breast. I felt a mass as big as an orange. There were also glands in her armpit that hadn't been there before, when the first surgeon had examined her. Although I knew from my training that a breast cancer was difficult to feel in a breast that was lactating, being full with breast milk, this still seemed unusual. I felt that the mass had somehow 'manifested' in the intervening time. I was once again in the realms of quantum physics ... and its association to the awkward word 'magic' presented itself.

What had I to offer? Certainly, nothing from my medical background.

Over the previous few years, Ann and I had stepped more into unconventional areas of health and healing. I now recalled the work of Carl and Stephanie Simonton and the use of visualisation in cancer. Ann asked me if he could assist her with this. So, we put a mattress on the private side veranda of the house, and I induced Ann into a light hypnotic state. I then encouraged her to visualise the cancer, but she could not. Concerned, I then asked her to do the same with her defensive immune system cells, but again she could not. I gave her some visual ideas, but this made no difference. I was floored. She was unable to visualise – not just the cancer or her immune system, but anything.

The meeting between Ann and I was a meeting of minds. Highly trained as a clinical psychologist and psychotherapist, Ann was interested in exploring other modalities of healing. She had heard of me and had approached me regarding dreams. We hit it off and agreed to meet periodically to look at Ann's dreams, but this never eventuated. Instead, the meetings became conversations about health and healing from a psychological perspective, and the attraction grew.

One evening we were both at a private function given by one of the new alternative healing centres. Drinks in hand, we gravitated to a side room and sat talking in chairs facing each other. I found the intensity magnetic; it was based on conversation, but in a manner that was like making love. And Ann felt the same – she didn't need to say it.

When we first consummated our relationship, Ann became distressed and cried immediately afterward. I was surprised, but accommodating; mainly because I didn't know what else to do, as I had not experienced a response like this before. A day or so later, when we were chatting at the beach, she raised this issue and said she believed that now I wouldn't want to take the relationship any further. I admired her forthrightness, as I had from the onset. I replied that I had met many people with problems and that we all have them, but in her I saw someone prepared to confront them. Yet a vague doubt stayed with me even as I said the words, but not to be raised with her, as the relief on Ann's face with my response was obvious.

Maybe we just went too quickly and didn't cover the bases. There are still so many questions in my mind, although I am now accepting of what came to pass. We lived together and conceived Chaz immediately. She told me she wanted to give me a son. I had two daughters from my prior marriage and she had one from hers. We took risks and saw our relationship as an adventure. It was only later that I realised how much Ann was pushing me, wanting me to act on her behalf. It was a false sense of empowerment, but I didn't see it. I discovered that power is something I can be blind to.

When we moved to the hills region of Darlington, I decided to open our own centre, Avalon House, in West Perth. The relationship with Ann had distanced me from the Jungian community; I had crossed an unspecified boundary. I saw the Jungians as anachronistic and that there were new vistas opening in other therapeutic and transpersonal areas. I wanted to be part of this changing landscape and, with Ann now present, my close relationships became more varied and eclectic. The senior Jungians disapproved, as they had about the relationship from its inception, when I had been questioned about it from the perspective of professional boundaries – an excuse to be critical and judgmental, I considered.

I now saw myself firmly in the area of depth psychology and psychotherapy, so I was surprised when I received a letter from the Medical Board about a complaint they had received that I was 'advertising' my services. The surprise was that I felt myself to be a long way from the medical community and now exploring other therapy modalities. I had opened Avalon and attracted others to join me, but none were medical in the early stages. I was interviewed in the daily paper about my interests, and this was the source of the complaint by an unknown medical practitioner.

I replied, but still they sanctioned me. I realised then that these institutions have long arms – "controlling tentacles" is the phrase I actually thought of at the time.

This would not be the only time I was to experience this sort of judgement and, of course, the source of the complaint remained unknown. I began to realise that being registered as a practitioner somehow stifled the expression of my status and growing experience as a medical doctor. It reinforced the vague sanctioning I was receiving from the Jungians. But all this was easily forgotten when the Medical Board sanction was a wrap on the knuckles; I was free to continue relatively unabated, though now a little more watchful and careful.

However, I knew I might now either become or already be a marked man with my apparently controversial views, which were expressed in the newspaper interview that had led to the complaint.

Avalon House had now been in operation nearly two years and was starting to be noticed. Up to that stage, there were two other similar centres in operation, but they were distinctly alternative. Ours was different: We now boasted medical practitioners, psychologists, and physiotherapists in addition to the various alternative therapists, meditation teachers, and yoga practitioners. As well as consultations and therapeutic practice, I had formed an association with academia that spawned fledgling educational courses in the healing arts.

The Jungian community now felt as distant as the medical one, although the recent brush with the

Medical Board reminded me that, whilst I was a registered Jungian analyst and medical practitioner then, there was a certain care and responsibility that accompanied registration. Many years later, my questioning of this was to create a vision that the whole area of registration requires serious examination and possible renewal itself. Issues of power, as well as sex, are poorly negotiated and remain tools to be used and abused by those in authority, I came to realise.

Ann sat on the floor of the centre; it was her custom, so I joined her. She was in the early stages of pregnancy. Asha had been conceived as she was finishing breastfeeding Chaz, so this pregnancy was unplanned. She had been breastfeeding him for a year when she developed inflammation in the same breast that was later to become cancerous. We decided to stop breastfeeding; the inflammation settled, but Asha snuck through the gap: A charmed child.

Ann wanted to go away for an extended break. Why now? I was both anxious and angry. We still had all the responsibilities of the centre and our house; the finances were improving, but they were not at break-even point. Ann was still practising, supporting the centre and their finances, and she wanted to go away! I felt she was being self-indulgent, but that was a justification for me because, deep down, I felt the plaintiveness in her voice. But it did not reach beyond the betrayal I now felt. I had seen something similar in her when we first met, after our first lovemaking, and would see it again. But on this occasion, I ignored it as other pressures of reality caved in on us. She agreed to stay.

It was a mistake: I should have let her go. I know

that now. The cancer somehow started when she had the breast inflammation, and even that association remains of professional and academic interest. I was having a tryst with someone from the community that had grown up around the centre at the time. Ann and I had an 'open' relationship and this was above board; it involved the three of us, on occasion. But later I was to discover that this affected her deeply. Was I being naïve or just plain cruel?

Beyond the challenges the centre would raise about therapy and healing, there were the social and community dimensions. These grew up around the practices and educational services. We both fostered and explored these, with the risks and unknowns they presented. The boundaries were different to those of formal health disciplines and academia, and challenged us in many ways.

I was well aware of this as a potential professional provocation; it was something I had confronted with the Jungians, although they had a covert community where the boundaries were different to the supposed professional standards, even if somewhat disguised. This duplicity I now know to be present in all such institutions, even the medical profession, and is the source of much hypocrisy. I hated it then and I hate it still.

This was all no surprise to me at the time; Jung himself had maintained such distinctions, even if covertly. Ever the man to keep a professional public persona, Jung maintained much secrecy over his private life. Yet it was rife with what might be considered 'transgressions', although the community itself was keen to protect him and his work. In this respect, I saw myself not dissimilar to Jung. However, times had changed and I was more public with mine; ultimately this more cavalier approach did not work in my favour.

The actual progression of the illness itself witnessed the demise of Avalon House. For a few months, things seemed to go on as normal in our family, but then the cancer started to break through the skin and manifest openly. We were to enter a new stage and were relatively unprepared. Up until that time I had maintained the centre and my practice but, with Ann not working, the financial strains were showing and the gaps opening up.

The community was at a relative loss in how to deal with the illness; they did their best, but Avalon was still in its early stages. Even so, a lot was learned by all involved. Maybe one of Ann's gifts was for the future of these people, myself included. However, I felt the strain and started the process of dissembling the centre. In my own mind, it would close and I would walk away from the venture, never to visit a project like this again. Or so I thought at the time.

Almost as an aside: Ian now shows me this written section above and I feel sick, even with myself. There is a level where it is bland, rather like writing in the third person. Has Ian done this, or has he accurately portrayed the emotional distance I had – and maybe still have – from these events? But it wasn't like that at all. In between the lines written is an emotional roller coaster of sickness, pain and despair that is difficult to describe. I watched Ann's slide toward death, slowly and inexorably. It was painful for her, and painful to watch. I slid into death with her and awoke alive; but alone.

It is only now I can begin to imagine fully what it would have been for her. I felt at the time that I was so wrapped in my narcissistic worldview that I had little time to empathise with what Ann was experiencing. I felt gutted, ashamed, and guilty. I found a dark emotion and judgement, and I felt it. Even now, I feel that many observers – maybe most – may not see beyond this; although I fully appreciate why this is so, it set me apart and still does.

At this point, Kennan expressed some confusion in the various threads that were emerging in the story. Although he had almost vowed that he would never again be involved in anything like Avalon House, it was a current possibility, although in a different context. He now wonders whether he had thrown the baby out with the bathwater over the intervening years.

Part of his explanation for this was that, with Ann's illness, the community aspect had tended to shift from the centre to their hillside home, so he came to believe that developing a community from a centre was not possible. What he was now beginning to realise was that he had it the wrong way around; that the centre evolved from the community and its needs. It is only recently he has started to revise what such a centre may look like.

Kennan explained to me that these ramifications were wide and also contained other elements that he had yet to recount. Instead, he felt he wanted to keep the focus on Ann's illness and death to see where that took the narrative. He also, at this point, made a wry comment about now recognising why, out of all the possible options, that it was Jane's story he told.

I asked: "Why?"

"Because it is also about birth, sex and death,' he replied, 'but with a different outcome."

There had been indications of all this in various ways. Kennan had indicated some initial challenges sexually in the relationship with Ann, and that they had mutually adopted an open one that was not defined by fidelity. I asked further about this and he was revealing, but he demurred in this account, telling me that such information might be open for discussion in workshops and retreats, but not for the general public in a book.

Kennan further explained that Ann and he had adopted an open view of their relationship in the context of themselves as explorative professionals, as well as in the immediate community that surrounded it. But this honesty and patency was not without a price.

With Ann's death, Kennan was to experience condemnation – indirectly of course – from the wider professional community, and even to be held somehow responsible for her death. This experience was to traumatise Kennan deeply. It was evident in the way he recounted some of condemnations to me personally (and which I have chosen not to recount), and how the broader professional community reacted. There was a moral self-righteousness and resistance to change that masked deeper murky factors, such as professional and personal envy, even jealousy. Yet this was all still to come, although the seeds are present here. However, this was not out in the open; something he came to term as 'social sorcery'.

Kennan also brought my attention to a sociological factor that had since been largely superseded. At the time he was forging the centre, there was a broad interest in Eastern mysticism, as Westerners became aware of their impoverishment in the spiritual fields. One so-called guru who attracted a lot of attention was a man referred to as Bhagwan Shree Rajneesh, later to change his name to Osho. The reason for this interest was that the community that surrounded Osho had a primarily therapeutic focus, and sexual liberation was also a strong feature.

Therapists at Kennan's centre were sometimes of this persuasion. Both Ann and Kennan were attracted to many elements of Osho's teaching, so it was somewhat inevitable that they would be tarred with the same brush. Anxious to clarify this themselves, they arranged to visit Osho's ashram in India after Ann was diagnosed, but before she became ill and chose not to go.

Initially reluctant to go alone, Kennan found himself on the plane a couple of months before Ann's death. She had insisted he go, as she had good support. He also suspected that she knew it was part of his future, but not hers. One evening she effectively said as much, also saying that Kennan would also have to sell their hillside home and give up practice.

Well, he was on his way to India, the house would sell in the months after her death, but it would take many years before he gave up practice. But all came to pass.

The weeks Kennan spent at the Rajneesh ashram had a deep and enduring impact on him. Kennan returned to Australia a changed man. But by this stage Ann was palpably ill; it was not only just local and apparent in her breast; she was also weak and she – the woman he knew – had effectively 'left' her body. The remaining few weeks after he returned – before her death – took on the appearance of a drama for others, but not for either Ann or Kennan.

I asked Kennan if he was disappointed with the course of action Ann took?

No, he accepted and endorsed it. Partly because it was her choice, and partly because he recognised his profession had little to offer. In fact, the thought of surgery and chemotherapy horrified them both and was not considered an option from an early stage, a view their surgeon friend also endorsed. Instead,

Ann opted for alternative approaches of various sorts. However, this was not systematic and somewhat of a roller coaster, in Kennan's opinion.

What had impressed Kennan was that Ann had been unable to visualise the cancer and, indeed, that her imagination in this mode was seemingly absent. Kennan was and is a voracious dreamer and he had then assumed all people could see imagery in the way he did. This was reinforced when he read her diaries some weeks after her death. She had left them for him, he deduced. When he read her dreams, he saw how she had not connected them with her daily reality in any meaningful way. And, in fact, he discovered that for someone who so eschewed the victim role, Ann was ultimately someone who played the part to the full. He was also able to see the unknown patterns that led to her illness, and they horrified him.

I am now aware that I have structured this chapter in the third person, rather than in dialogue. I hadn't noticed it when I started, but I now reflect that we didn't really dialogue; Kennan was immersed in the account, so I have simply recorded this and relayed it in this way. But I also suspect it is to somehow give it a little more distance, even emotionally; the interesting effect for me is that it has started to get a more mythic flavour in this process.

A further point, if I dare: Kennan did not make the final connection between Jane's story and what has been revealed about Ann, so maybe it is my turn to come to a couple of conclusions! The first is that Jane was able to visualise her nemesis; to give it 'shape', so to speak. In this, Kennan was able to join her in seeing the vision; how much of this was psychic, even magical? Also, how much did it occur because of any psycho-erotic tension between them? Lastly, Jane immediately ritualised this with a drama that, in and of itself, led to the change, the healing.

Although Kennan will, and has, come to all this in his work, it is simply that I noted that they were not embedded in the account of that time. I then wonder how much this writing process is providing these connections for him, and so healing him. And I wonder how much the roles have reversed in this part of his story and that I have become the healer?

Back to Kennan ...

> The ashram was based on the cult of the Guru; that is the Indian way. It was not familiar to me, but I could accept it while I was there. What impressed me, apart from Osho himself, was the organisation of the ashram. The therapy was embedded in the community, and the boundaries of this were well organised. I could see that this was not the case in my work back in Australia. There the community had developed from the centre, and I now associated this with failure.
>
> When I returned home, the community was supporting Ann and my young family. It was also supporting me personally. As my working days unravelled into a void, to be only addressed when necessary, the support of Ann and her death was foremost in my mind. My care of the children was certainly not ideal in that period, but there were several people, particularly women in the community, who helped fill that role.
>
> Some were also later to fill my bed. This gave me relief at several levels and made me question where sex and death were related.
>
> I subsequently found this was common to many men in their middle years whose partners were dead or dying of cancer, particularly of the breast. I also saw how the broader community condemned such

behaviour and that I would be similarly judged. But the association of this with responsibility for Ann's death was a surprise, though contained a truth that I would only unravel over time: because at some deep level, I was responsible, and I knew it.

Life moved on. Avalon House had closed and my practice now occupied a room at home again. I had moved from our hillside home in Darlington to be closer to the Osho community in Fremantle, which gave me needed support without judgement and also offered a sense of a life beyond.

One friend saw me sitting depressed on the back step of the house when Ann was nearly passed away. He was an ex-policeman and he provoked me into a fight; a fight I would always lose. Marty was bigger, stronger, and better equipped than me, but we fought to a standstill; something he had planned, no doubt. Seated on the grass afterwards, he then went inside and came back with two large open bottles of beer. We drank in silence, but I felt much, much better. A perplexed audience had silently witnessed the whole scene, although we combatants had been far from quiet.

This was also how my sexuality was now conducted. There was no presumption of a relationship; that was the nature of the Osho community. If one matured from the intimacy, that was fine, but at this time it was usually transient. Ironically, it attracted into my orbit women from outside the immediate community, as if the sex were a magnet to it. I began to understand the relationship between sexuality and healing, as Marty had made me see it with aggression.

During this period, I had no contact from the

medical profession. I hardly expected it. If I was to have any, I imagined it would be the result of a complaint. Nor did any of the Jungian analysts contact me, except one brief phone call from a colleague in another state. At this time, I received, via a girlfriend's receipt of them, anonymous letters of condemnation and judgment. These 'poison pen' letters were from someone with an apparent feminist inclination of a particular variety, who would not identify themselves, but who displayed a strange ambivalence in the condemnation; it felt like attraction. Marty, with his background, had subsequently been able to determine the source and the picture fitted my prior assessment.

I had decided that I could no longer be a Jungian analyst and resigned, something I had been considering for many months anyway. There was enough flack for the organisation to make this resignation easy to accept. But I decided to retain my medical registration, as I felt that it was unlikely I would continue as a psychotherapist in the immediate future, but could conduct some medical practice for income. Instead, I made plans to move to the south coast.

I was not sure how I felt about the above meeting with Kennan and the account that unfolded. I had a strange sense of being in a void and a little outside of time. The people and activities of the café that normally would attract at least my occasional attention were not noticed at all. We did not stop for a coffee refill or a piss break. At the end of our meeting, we parted in relative silence following a hug.

Kennan had told me that we could now discuss, in more detail, the three-year period that had led to this time and that we would do it when next we met. I was happy with that, and it did settle one query for me. But there were so many loose ends in this part of the account. And if there were for me, I could only guess about how confused and maybe lost Kennan had felt in the midst of this.

There are also two levels of secrecy in what we had shared. Firstly, I felt there was much, much more that Kennan could have shared with me, but chose to retain. As he stated, some of this he felt he could share in other settings, such as workshops and retreats, although maybe in limited and instructive ways. And I am sure, over time, were we to continue, these other implied stories would surface between us with full emotional vigour.

There were also some he shared that he asked not to be committed to writing, as well as some that did not receive that caveat, but which I have chosen not to commit to print. This all amounts to a strange and varied mixture. Within Kennan there is an almost insistently overwhelming desire for revelation, almost confession, which I suspect only the years have tempered. But he believed and still believes that such revelation is necessary and important. And he particularly feels this in the health and healing fields, especially on the subject of sexuality, as well as their interconnection.

But Kennan is also now more experienced and cognisant of some of the boundaries that need to be in place for this to be effective, creative, and not counter-productive. Some of this I am sure he learnt from his experience of Osho and time in the ashram.

But mostly it is born of his own painful experience.

Eight

Kennan felt that it is only now, a generation later, that he is picking up on some of the significant threads of his life that had existed in the three years prior to Ann's death. Such was the shadow this event placed on his life and work. He was also quick to point out that they lived at a time when, rightly or wrongly, there was more openness and experimentation in the therapeutic area than exists now.

Kennan feels this more adventurous time has passed, although I know he hopes for it again in the future, even if not for himself. Initially, he thought it was because of the 'baby and bathwater' experience; that Ann's death had obscured and blocked such adventure. But now he recognises that increasing institutionalisation, political and legal control, and corporate interference are the main reasons. These were to become significant factors in his choice to cease being a medical practitioner that, in many ways, paralleled his departure from Jungian analysis and formed a clear psychological pattern in him.

That departure from practice in itself has been another grief, he informed me. With nearly forty years in medical practice of one sort or another, it would always take more than a couple of drinks at a bar, or a period of leave, to bury the experience and move on. I asked him how long it did take. He told me it was about three years before he felt that he had even resurfaced.

"In fact, it wasn't until a bout of pneumonia that I could honestly say I am no longer grieving the loss of the medical profession in my life. I have also come to see how much I had engineered the departure, so that it could be final, complete. I also know I can never go back into medical practice, certainly as it is now. And, somewhat ironically, but maybe predictably, I feel that the final shards of the grief for Ann were apparent and available to be pulled out. I also have a sense of being 'back on track' and that Ann would approve. I do recall her telling me I'd have to leave practice. I thought at the time that she meant therapeutic practice, but now I see it was medical."

"You think the pneumonia was significant?" I asked. Because, of course, I already knew about this.

"Yes," was the quick reply, "I certainly do! Infectious disease seems to be my lot in life, some would say my karma; but it is so. You'll see that in what is yet to come, as well as the problems I had as an infant and young child, if you recall. The pneumonia didn't surprise me when it happened."

"What actually did happen? We didn't really discuss this in detail at the time."

"Well, I had just arrived back in Australia from a trip to Bali, as you know, and I had picked up a cold. I presumed it was this, because my wife had it too, but as she recovered mine just progressed. I had temperatures, felt like death, and had an awful and very painful cough. I presumed it was viral, because whilst there was muck in my lower chest mainly on the right, the small amount of sputum I was bringing up didn't seem bacterial in nature. So, I just managed it symptomatically. It lasted several weeks. In hindsight, I think it was a SARS infection, and maybe some sort of psychic precursor to the arrival of Covid a few years later.

"Yet it was the psychic side that intrigued me. All the issues about having been a medical practitioner for so long, and the choice to no longer be one three years before, simply fell away. And I know this because the dreams about medical activities stopped at this time. As I started to recover, I started to feel a vitality and enthusiasm that I could trace back to the days of the centre and the years with Ann. But it also felt like she was no longer around; or if she was, it was not in the same way."

Kennan told me, on previous encounters, that his own doctor, James, had always considered he had a post-traumatic stress disorder – PTSD. This had arisen as a result of a stress-related illness he had developed in the last year of his medical practice, as well as his discussions with James about his use of alcohol for this.

Alcohol had become an increasing issue over the years following Ann's death. What had been a social and sometimes therapeutic habit became a problematic one. Kennan talked with James about this, particularly with the stress illness he had over the year before leaving practice. James always maintained that Kennan was not an alcoholic, but had a PTSD problem that "drove him to drink". Being a relative specialist in addictions, he believed James ought to know, although others might have considered otherwise. To Kennan, it is all a moot point. James also felt that a severe illness he was to develop following Ann's death was a significant historical factor in the overall traumatic pattern.

As the world is now wrestling with the Covid crisis, it would be seductive to link this infective experience to the present and bypass the intervening few years, but I knew this would be a mistake. I could sense in the alcohol story that the pneumonia was probably going to lead him into some difficult and unknown territory. I did not want to lose track of this period when instead Kennan was leading me into the future.

I reminded him of his promise that we would cover the years prior to Ann's death that he had made at our previous meeting. He smiled and, after a deep and conscious breath, he began to recount that period.

Prior to meeting Ann, I had felt somewhat isolated

from the Jungian community. I started to realise this toward the end of my training and had doubts about continuing with such a close liaison, even whether I should complete the analytic training. But I had too much invested in it. I had burnt my bridges with psychiatry; I no longer considered general medical practice as an option; my social network and relationship of the time were embedded in the Jungian community, and my psychotherapy practice was still reliant on it.

There were features of the Jungian professional community that I questioned. It was itself isolated in the broader healthcare community and comprised individuals who had emerged through the analytic ranks, and who were sometimes of questionable professional standards, yet were now in positions of power. There was a kind of spiritual arrogance about being Jungian, almost to the point that Jung himself was deified. Certainly, his psychology was, as espoused locally. In effect, Jungian psychology was becoming anachronistic and out of phase with recent therapeutic trends; in need of healing, I might add.

I have already drawn attention to the significance and influence of Osho, which seemed pertinent to the concerns I held, so a closer association with that community added to the discontent. As did the blossoming of other therapeutic approaches that rivalled Jung in a more modern context, which the Jungians tended to judge with disdain, whilst I wanted to explore them. Also, the influence of the sixties, psychedelic drugs and the 'psychonauts' – often doctors and psychologists – was still palpable.

Ann came from a disciplined psychological background, practiced as a psychotherapist, and had trained in a discipline that then rivalled Jung. It seemed a marriage made in heaven; except we never did get married! The other marked similarity between us was that we were both questioning our psychotherapeutic disciplines and saw ourselves in the wider transpersonal and human potential movements that were flourishing at the time.

In a way, these factors defined our coming together and relationship. When we sat back a little later, we realised how dissimilar our personal backgrounds were; although within them were similar problems and traumas that had brought us into the therapeutic arena in the first place. Also, we were now relatively unpopular in our respective therapeutic training communities, each of which would blame the partner from the other camp for having led their respective acolytes away from the fold. However, some from our broader respective communities, most of our clients, and certainly the Osho community, would follow us with the changes we undertook.

None of this worried Ann and me. When pregnant with Chaz, I decided to formalise the changes and develop a more eclectic professional centre called Avalon House in West Perth, with Ann's support. On her part, Ann engineered a move to the hills and a rambling property on a couple of acres in Darlington that would be an extension of the centre for workshops, as well as being our residence. The vision was starting to take shape.

The stresses were proportional to the accelerated changes. Chaz was born at home. The erotic liaisons that had unsettled Ann prior to Asha's conception had emerged from and were engineered into a social, psychological and sexual setting that was part of our community. People frequently stayed at our house and this became more formalised when we moved to the hills. I felt in my element, but it wasn't apparent to me at the time how much Ann was following my lead, whilst simultaneously encouraging and pushing me forward.

In hindsight, there was an experience that occurred just prior to our move to the hills that should have alerted us both, myself particularly. I had always had a psychic tendency as a child, but in my schooling, this had largely been displaced, or more accurately repressed by a disciplined academic approach. Yet I remained subliminally eccentric, wild at times, creative at others. People were attracted to me, whilst I knew others saw me in devilish guise. I was a relative pioneer and innovator.

Yet many of these qualities I had downplayed and marginalised over the years since school. My desire for success in the world often made such features inconvenient or even disruptive. This was another place where alcohol came in. As I have already said, at a very early stage in my career I realised that dipping into the doctor's bag, or using the prescription pad for myself, would be a literally fatal error on my part. I thereafter never considered it. But alcohol made for social adjustment and stress release, as well as some tolerable acceptance of these other personality features to others, particularly when it came to sexual expression.

On this particular night, I had finished work and gone out drinking. This, in itself, was unusual. My alcohol intake was usually domestic in the family setting or social situations that extended from these. But on this occasion, it followed a game of squash with a friend. I recall that I arrived home in a playful, but slightly drunken state, to find Ann breastfeeding Chaz in front of an open fire in a room of the house we rarely used together. This heightened the atmosphere between us, as I felt in a time out of time, so to speak.

Of course, Ann was more than a little psychic herself. Her comment about "giving you a son" and immediately following it with conception – in fact that same night – was at the very least profoundly intuitive. I was to realise in the years following her death that it was this quality in her that most attracted me.

On this occasion, Ann was more serious. I sat down and she asked me some searching questions. These were not personal, so I entered into the spirit of the dialogue and, combined with the alcohol, found myself in a dreamy state when answering. Then the tone moved; she started to ask questions about herself and Chaz, but it wasn't until afterwards that I digested what had happened.

Ann asked me how many more children we would have together. I knew prior that she wanted two more, and ideally they would be another boy and a girl. But I was in a state and 'saw' only one, a girl. I told her. She then asked about our future together. I answered that it would be for a while, with our daughter, but I saw nothing after that. She challenged me: Did this mean we would break up? I didn't know; all I could see was blank – and it then became dark.

Kennan told me that he only fully recalled this encounter the next day when he was sober. In fact, he didn't remember it at all until Ann brought the subject up. This surprised him; he didn't think he had had that much to drink. Then he realised that he had been in a trance state, an altered state of consciousness, and this is why he had apparently forgotten.

However, there was another factor here that he had not taken full credit of: Alcohol. For many years, Kennan saw this as an incidental in the event, or at the most to have facilitated the process. He did not see how much the alcohol had itself induced the altered mental state he found himself in, something he was to slowly discover in his shamanic researches later. He was also to experience it directly in the disturbing last year of his practice days, and to be associated with writing a book on the Anglo-Saxon runes. He was finally to face its impact in the years between the SARS pneumonia and his illness immediately prior to the emergence of Covid.

Ann had then used him in a divinatory capacity, asking him questions, as one would a fortune-teller. Kennan was shocked when he realised all of this and that his loss of memory was because of the state he had entered. He was only recently speculated on these so-called alcoholic memory blackouts as having a deeper significance; a doorway psychically, a kind of portal.

As we sat in silence, Kennan was pensive. It was almost as if he had forgotten the story. As I asked him a little more, he made connections between the darkness he saw and the cancer. This was because, when Ann actually died, he experienced passing into that darkness – a void – and when he came out, she had stopped breathing. It was at this point in time that he now realised that the cancer had probably started, and that the conversation they had on the floor at the centre – about Ann needing to go away – actually happened as a consequence. Maybe this was this event that had led to her request to go away?

Kennan was pale, beads of sweat on his forehead, dreamy eyes gazing into an unknown distance. He already felt a sense of responsibility regarding her death, yet now it seemed to be more significant. It was associated with the state he was in – that he was later to recognise as shamanic – and hence the deeper sense of responsibility. But as we talked, he also recalled Jane's experiences and the vision of the spider. Somehow Jane had 'seen' this and negotiated her potential death. Ann did not, and he was only to realise this on the veranda when she was not able to visualise the cancer. And it was only now, as we talked, that he was to fully realise all this.

He looked at me, unblinking, with tears now rolling down his cheeks. This exchange reinforced my earlier deductions, written prior to this episode. Yet I also felt privileged; I was watching – involved in – healing in action.

The deeper parallels with Ann and Jane were about sex and death. In Ann's case, birth and death were very strongly associated, as they were also with Jane, indirectly. As we discussed this further, Kennan saw that we could simply follow an intellectual analysis and he then shied away, instead focusing on the associations of birth, sex, and death. Elsewhere he had explored this pattern in his writing, even nominating it as the Great Cycle of Existence. Here and now in our discussion, it was taking on a greater and more personal meaning. My suspicion was that this would spawn a further creative exploration of the pattern at some future time.

Kennan's thinking moved to the issue of responsibility. With Ann, it was as if he was taking responsibility for her, and that she was asking him to. This was not unlike a therapeutic relationship and what can occur between the therapist and client, but here the situation was different. It was also deeper in the sense that it touched areas beyond intellectual appreciation and more suited to the psychic world and the imagination.

Maybe this is why Ann had encouraged Kennan – unbeknownst to him at the time – to undertake this responsibility. Maybe also he had missed an opportunity and that the initial pattern of their meetings, around dreams and dream interpretation, was directing them toward a therapeutic relationship of sorts, even if somewhat shamanic. But he had not seen that at the time, possibly because of his own needs, and also because he was not yet experienced enough.

Nor had Kennan seen all this on the veranda, where she was possibly asking him to do the visualisation for her … because she couldn't? Nor again in the interaction in front of the fire. Although divining, did he have an opportunity to change the pattern then? Could he have taken what he 'saw' and imagined it further to a different path and outcome? In the shamanic sense, was Ann asking for 'retrieval of her soul'? And when he was drawn into the dark void at her death, was this an opportunity to retrieve his?

The mood was getting sombre. I made a decision to change the conversation and asked Kennan directly what Avalon House had achieved, other than the difficulties described to date. Because, it seemed to me that, excluding Ann's death, the centre was innovative, creative, and breaking many moulds: He agreed. Although he had explained the origins of the centre in personal terms, I asked him specifically about this more philosophical perspective:

"Well," he answered, "as you can see it was mainly conceived as an extension of our therapeutic explorations. Both of us were comfortable with our respective trainings, but we weren't happy with some of the restrictions that this brought about."

"What restrictions?" I asked.

"There are the obvious ones that go along with any institutionalisation. Then there are the ones that are due to time; that the approaches we used were becoming anachronistic, and themselves in need of renewal. We also saw in that period that a more eclectic and multi-disciplined approach was necessary.

"This all brought in other factors. The main one we experienced and had to negotiate was the social or community side of what we were doing. Initially, we were a bit isolated, although watched from a safe distance with apparent interest. We also developed our own following and had to appreciate, understand and deal with that. As you can see to date, that wasn't always successful."

"So, you didn't entertain something more mind-and-body?"

"Not initially. As you can see, I was miles away from modern medicine at this time. However, Ann was very interested in bodily approaches to psychotherapy, and this interested us both as we progressed. We also had various practitioners become involved who were of this inclination. So, I started to take an interest myself and reflect this back onto my medical knowledge and experience, although it didn't enter my practice; I remained a psychotherapist and analyst through and through, at this time.

"Then, via Avalon House's community – one a previous client and another from the Osho community – two medical practitioners showed an interest in being involved as general practitioners and therapists. This then set us apart from the other two centres that were then operating. It also stayed with me as a possibility with the centre's demise; there was a lot of common ground between modern medicine, therapy, and alternative approaches yet to be negotiated.

"Of course, in the present era, this has been somewhat appropriated by the medical profession, though not at the explorative depth we were negotiating. Such that alternative health approaches that are either acceptable somehow in mainstream, or which are proven to be effective, are now called complementary; although this is still judged from the standards of modern western medicine, and I think that is a mistake."

"Why?" I was quick to ask.

"Because it is not as if the medical profession is being open-minded and creative; it is effectively just dealing with a situation it can't avoid any longer. So, we have a mixed bag of disciplines and approaches that are acceptable, as they now cannot be excluded. This is because the so-called evidence-based approach that medicine has adopted means that some inclusions, which may otherwise be dismissed, now have to be accepted. Acupuncture is a good example of this. Now you have medical practitioners training as acupuncturists and practising it with rebates, although not usually accepting of the philosophy it stems from, and subsequently marginalising probably better and more experienced alternative practitioners. Philosophy, in this respect, is a reflection of the psychospiritual and, as you now know, I see this as indispensable to any true healing approach.

"Then you have awkward evidence, such as amphetamines being successful in the treatment of attention deficit disorders. The way this is dealt with is by marginalising – even within the profession – practitioners who utilise this treatment, as well as now making it almost impossible to prescribe anyway!

"But maybe I'm getting off the track. The whole alternative-complementary debate is a big and very contemporary issue. It is not one at the time we were getting involved in directly; we were simply exploring therapeutic options in all manner of disciplines and ways. Our doctors were just facilitating this, as I was limited in what I could and was – then – prepared to offer; although I did prescribe and medically investigate my clients, if needed."

I commented: "I'm sure we'll return to the 'Complementary and Alternative Medicine' or CAMS debate later, but it seems to me your comments have some issues of the present in them?"

"Yes, that's true. At the time, this sort of work had not got to the point where the profession felt threatened in the way it now does, so we were just being experimental and relatively adventurous."

"Such as when?"

"Well, this was more confined to our educational approaches."

"Ah." I pricked my ears up. "I recall you had that dimension in the centre as well. How did that work?"

"Mainly through the association I had with a colleague who worked in the area of professional development. He was an academic and not a medical doctor. He had a significant and active interest in private teaching and education in the health arena, and I was keen to learn as well."

"Learn what, exactly?"

"Learn to be a teacher. In medicine and therapy, I came to see that teaching and education are an important function, though often minimised and now commonly dismissed. I had used an educative approach in medicine in my general practice days, and certainly it was – and is – a significant component in psychotherapy. But, at that time, my approach to any teaching was fairly ad hoc and informal in style. I needed teaching myself!

"I only realised that this was what I was doing in a progressive way over the ensuing years. At that time, with my colleague Rafael's direction, I simply wanted to set up some educational programmes as an extension of the centre's practice and therapy functions. So, I conducted various seminars and workshops: I say 'I' because Rafael was not actively involved here, and other practitioners only became so as we progressed.

"I enjoyed these programmes, and they added a really creative and explorative dimension to what we were doing. I recall a workshop that I thought up: I used light trance states and played particular pieces of evocative music. In these states, I provided what is known as a 'journey', which was basically an imaginative exercise. Then, after coming out of the trance at the end of the music, I asked the participants to draw or crayon any images they experienced. I was astounded at the similarity of imagery. On one occasion four of the six participants had almost identical pictures. There are many ways you could reason and interpret this, but it opened up lines of therapeutic inquiry that were fascinating.

"I also worked with an astrologer for a period. We took client's dreams and matched my interpretations with what are called astrological transits. We were both intrigued by the resonance between the two approaches, as were the participants. Unfortunately, he and I were too intuitively inclined to be able to organise and progress what we had discovered in any sort of formal way."

"And how did you medical practitioners get along with each other in Avalon?"

"One thing that has always impressed me about medical practitioners is their incredible reluctance to talk about how they manage their patients. They talk about medical cases and investigations, but actually about how they conduct a consultation? Very little. We were a little better at Avalon, and the alternative practitioners even more so."

"Can you explain this attitude amongst medical practitioners?"

"Fear of exposure, I guess? Only by exploring a case in this manner would you find out what was behind it at the personal level, I suspect."

"Okay, back to the centre's approach."

"Well, we did discuss cases informally, with the usual professional safeguards and caveats around this, of course. But we also engaged with each other therapeutically."

I was intrigued: "Meaning?"

"We had sessions with each other. I experienced bodywork, yoga therapy, primal therapy, breathwork … you name it, I did it. So did Ann, as well as most of the others. We explored the outcome of these sessions and the therapeutic implications.

Sexual exploration was not off our radar, either. I used to invite visiting therapists to any workshop I did and get them to show their art, usually by working on individuals there and – if appropriate – getting them to learn and work on each other. All very varied, as you can see!

"I am very drawn to the discipline of alchemy and, in hindsight, I think we were conducting a collective alchemical experiment. However, and extending the alchemical metaphor, maybe the vessel containing the constituents was broken before the experiment was completed!"

I knew he was referring to Ann's death here.

"So, it was all a mess; confused and – to some – left in a dirty and ugly state, before anything really creative could come out of it.

"I suppose that is one reason that, at the time, I decided to simply close the door on the whole experience and, as I've already said, I think that in hindsight I threw the baby out with the bathwater. Because, even as I recount it now, there was so much we did and explored, and so much further we might have taken it all.

"Or maybe it was just a stage in a larger alchemical experiment, even up to and including my life. It is interesting how so many of the strands have re-emerged in the intervening years at different times and often under different guises, as I'm sure we are exploring here. It is only in the last couple of years that the various strands seem to be coming together in some sort of meaningful whole and, ironically, I felt I needed to leave the medical profession for this. This was never the intention … at a conscious level, that is!"

I had the feeling that the process of discussion and exploration that we were undertaking was helping Kennan to gain further clarity, and I was pleased. He seemed very isolated at times, limited with friends who could meet and challenge him, as well as travelling companions on his journey. I would return to this point, and made a mental note, as such. The experience of and in Avalon House had burnt him deeply, if I can be excused a further alchemical metaphor.

I also had my own feelings to contend with. The account that I was trying to put together, since Kennan's year in psychiatry, seemed to have become a bit of a blur. I think the account of that particular year unsettled me more than I had realised to date. It had certainly taken me well beyond my personal experience in medical practice and exposed me to ethical patterns that may be continuously operating, but about which I was previously unaware.

This was, in itself, disturbing for and to me. In this respect, I had lost some of my objectivity and critical positioning with respect to Kennan, and was emotionally walking more with him. Paradoxically, there were times when the flow between us seemed to oscillate and even reverse, which might not have been the case without this disturbance. I had much to consider.

I wondered whether I should rewrite these last few chapters, as a consequence. However, I ultimately decided not to. It would have been disingenuous and also difficult for me to form the objectivity that would be required to create the tension in our dialogue, which I felt had permeated the earlier chapters.

I had become profoundly affected by Kennan's plight and was empathising with him – considerably. I feel that the cyclic and flowing discourse is reflected in my writing, so maybe I was discovering another way of writing?

Nine

It took many hours to complete the burning. Kennan cast a strange image in the forest, dressed only in a black kaftan. He was in the most southerly location habitable, choosing to stay in an isolated shack following Ann's funeral. It was cold, bitterly so at times, but refreshing to the soul.

The funeral had been uneventful. One of their colleagues at Avalon was an ordained minister and he facilitated the service. Kennan recalled seeing Ann for the last time in the coffin prior to the service. It was inevitably a strange experience, but he felt it was important as some sort of ritual of closure that the children see their mother, too. Afterwards, on the way to the cremation, the driver, who was also Kennan's temporary host, began singing the pop song *I've Just Lost My Baby!* that came on the radio. His passenger – his wife – admonished him, but it seemed appropriate somehow to Kennan and the driver. A strange laughter resulted. This couple had been Ann's hosts in her final days. She had been offered a room there by the wife, who was a prior colleague of Ann's when Kennan was in India.

The tentacles from the past were also in operation around this end-game, Kennan told me with a wry smile. He added that a comment made by a female colleague after Ann's death sometime later confirmed for Kennan the erotic dimension of their relationship – told to him for reasons unknown but not difficult to ascertain. All sorts of levels of jealousy and retribution seemed to be floating around and Kennan felt he could almost see most of them in action, such was the power of his sight, except when they involved him though.

The drive down to the shack had been erratic, punctuated by a late pub dinner. Kennan simply wanted to get out of the city and so, assisted by two friends, he gathered the children up and set off immediately after the funeral. He felt that the chapter in his life that was closing very rapidly involved not only the loss of Ann, but also many associations that were present at the service.

Kennan was burning his books in the forest – these being diaries and other writings that had been accumulated over the years, centred round his analytic training and practice – the black kaftan he had bought in India whilst at the ashram. There was a white one that he would use at a later wedding – they were a matching pair. The books took four hours to burn completely. It seemed to him that all traces of his life to this point that could be examined, through any reading by others, needed to depart along with Ann's death.

After this, Kennan returned to their Darlington house. A strange period followed. The centre contained the shadow of what had occurred and went through its own slow demise. Many there Kennan would never see after it ultimately closed. He sold the hillside house and moved closer to the local Osho community in Fremantle that had supported him more emotionally during this period. He had hoped the centre's members would have provided this function, but this was not to be.

Leaving Avalon was, at one level, an easy thing to do. Kennan practised from his new home for a while, as his therapy and practice underwent a natural and inevitable contraction and revisioning process. Then he moved to the Osho community's communal house to work and be involved in their activities and meditations. In one way, this saved his life. He had a couple of health scares that, in hindsight, were probably more serious than he had considered at the time. But he didn't particularly care.

Being with the children was difficult, sometimes very difficult. The joys were intense, but too brief. Obviously too young to understand and with demands of their own, they taxed Kennan in emotional ways that were unfamiliar. His own moods fluctuated wildly, with sex and alcohol taking a regular part of his therapeutic regimen.

I found it difficult to follow Kennan during this period. It seemed disjointed in the relating, and I felt that relatively internal chaos was still present within him. Whilst I suspected this was due to the grief process in my own rather simplistic way, there was also a strange sense of time slipping and sliding around, even as we talked. It was as if Kennan was being carried by a tide, such that issues like his own health concerns became incidental or even irrelevant.

It was not that Kennan didn't care for the children. But this was strongly influenced by his emotional states and he simply followed these, giving up any clear expectation of 'getting it right' or 'doing it for the children'. If anyone approached him in that way they got short shrift, and most chose not to even try, he suspected. Rather, he fashioned his caring in the midst of the turmoil that had preceded Ann's death and was now following the three travellers like a deep, dark shadow.

And I noticed things with him now; such as less eye contact; frequent toilet breaks; no coffee refill, and certainly no smiling or jokes. Kennan was immersed in this period in a way that had a different quality than anything he had been like prior, even when describing and discussing Ann's illness and death. Our discussion here was minimal and certainly didn't explore extensions as before, like meaning and implications, or interpretations. He eschewed all such manner of discussion.

The mood lifted when Kennan related packing up and moving south and out of city life; maybe it was a lifesaver.

To my mind, the decision had been an easy one to make. I recall being in the kitchen one evening and looking at my children. I imagined them growing, something I had not done to date, and that they would need to go to school. A page was turning. I then felt I didn't want this to be in the city; in fact, I didn't want them to be brought up in the city at all. Then I asked myself the obvious rhetorical question: If I don't want them to live in the city, then why the hell am I living here?

The move was a matter of weeks after that question. Unable to find a rental, I purchased an old house in the town of Denmark in the Great Southern. I had a babysitter for the children after the move and commuted one week in two to Perth to earn a living, whilst developing a presence down south. Then, when life appeared to be settling into a rhythm, and the darkness lightened a little, I developed a fever.

Initially I thought this was just the flu. But it dragged on. There was a rhythm: I would have recovered somewhat in the morning, become lethargic toward lunchtime, and then tire in the afternoon. At night, my temperature would rise and I would start sweating. There were no other symptoms of note beyond those a fever produces, like joint pain, except a sharp pain at the tip of my right shoulder. I also lost a lot of weight.

I should have known then what this shoulder pain signified, but identifying a symptom in others was child's play compared with it happening to and in one's own body. I would get better at this recognition as time went on and I was to experience more illness, but at this time I was simply dismissive and put it down to an old shoulder injury.

Only later, when the cause of this illness was finally identified, would I make a complete sense of my symptoms then simultaneously eventually arrive at a more holistic understanding of illness and disease. I also began to wonder how any doctor could be truly effective as a practitioner without such an experience. It was a paradox that I would only resolve when I entered the strange world of shamanism in a more deliberate and conscious manner than I had hitherto.

But during this period the fevers did not abate. The local doctor did various exploratory blood tests. I had a distinct and strong pattern of an infective process, but with no obvious focus in any organ. Instead, the doctor determined I had a blood-borne infection. Various antibiotics were tried but with no success. Then, just as hospitalisation and further investigation was being considered, the fever abated.

Prior to this relief, during one bout of fever I had a vision. There was a succession of images; blood was pouring over the foreshore into the nearby Denmark river. There was a feeling of anguish and pain, but no clear images, just blood. I recounted this to my doctor; I trusted her, maybe more in this capacity than with my illness. She surprised me by telling me that a massacre had occurred there a hundred years before.

The local people had rounded up the aboriginal population and shot them on the foreshore. Those that survived, for whatever reason, were driven east out of the area for many miles. The medicine man, or shaman of the people, was then crucified on a tree next to a river that marked the territorial boundary as a warning to the others not to return.

And they didn't return.

I had been bemused by the lack of an aboriginal

presence when I first moved to Denmark, being only told there was a curse on the place. Then one day, whilst looking for a smallholding to buy, I talked with the elderly father of a real estate agent on an isolated farm many miles to the west:

"It was the epidemic." The man said this, in a matter-of-fact way, in response to my question as to why there was no aboriginal population in the area.

"What epidemic?" I asked.

"Well, it was the turn of the century. I was just a boy," he replied. "The flu came through and wiped them out."

At the time, I accepted this story with some further embellishment. Why should I think otherwise? Then my doctor's tale and explanation of my visionary experience made me revise what had really happened. It was a lead epidemic transmitted by rifles.

I was shocked, even in the midst of the illness. Something gnawed at me: If this was why I had the illness, then what was it telling me?

I recovered and forgot that question. I should not have because my alcohol intake now took on a different and more concerning pattern. I put this down to grief, but intuitively knew it was more than that, as I was over the main hurdle of Ann's death. It was now with alcohol excess that the visions would occur, when the psychic doors were ajar. I obviously was drawn to the visions, but why?

As the illness spontaneously subsided, almost as quickly as it had arisen, Kennan appraised his situation. He also moved out of town and, after a stay in a commune where he felt he put body and soul back together, he went to live in the regional town-cum-city of Albany and started medical practice again. This choice had emerged from local demand. Although he continued with some psychotherapy, the town lacked anyone of a more alternative disposition, so he provided this function in a general practice setting of his own making.

Albany was then an anachronism medically; maybe it still is, being set as it is in a culture that has slid a little behind modern time. The doctors had often gravitated there for various reasons other than medical practice, as there were little in the way of future career opportunities in the profession this far from the state capital. There was lifestyle, financial reward, and the management of the local hospital in a manner similar to Kalgoorlie. Except, at this time in Albany, there were no hospital residents: the resident general practitioners managed the show with the support of a couple of local specialists, plus a few who visited from the city periodically.

Kennan did not fit that mould. In fact, he was then the only doctor in practice to operate outside it. He reasoned that he had a small idiosyncratic practice and that the other doctors would not treat his patients the way he did and vice versa, so what was the point? Therefore, he remained out of the local system, with a few minor clashes on occasions, but essentially to keep his head down and create a practice of a more holistic orientation.

Holism to Kennan then was a descriptive word for his practice and not a life philosophy. But it emerged into his medical practice from his innate disposition, as well as his wide exposure to mental illness and psychological disturbance. Not only did he see that the mind and emotions must be considered in all illness, but that the various bodily systems interacted and were integrated as a fundamental unity. He saw this as a maturing position from the rather mechanical and overly scientific manner in which medicine is delivered in the modern era, and was repeatedly surprised that most other practitioners of experience did not come to a similar position.

Yet, as the years moved on, Kennan came to understand why other doctors did not. In many ways, their development as practitioners, and sometimes as people, ceased with qualification. Also, the practice and delivery of medicine as an art was increasingly submerged under scientific advances, technology, protocols, as well as the institutional outlook and controls that supported it. He maintained his head down stance, and quietly went about his business.

Kennan supported his practice with a nutritional and environmental orientation, both of which stemmed directly from his more advanced qualifications in physiology, being the science of the normal workings of the body. This extended to a counselling orientation and was supported by using treatment approaches, then and still controversial, that supported this new orientation.

For example, Kennan provided chelation therapy. Chelation is where one chemical reacts with others rather like a claw. In this respect, a specific chemical is used as a chelating agent, passed into the body through an intravenous infusion, and then it passes out in the urine as a natural consequence with what it claws in the process. The particular chemical used as a chelating agent specifically claws and removes chemically compliant poisons and heavy metals that have accumulated in the body that are considered responsible for a multitude of degenerative diseases, specifically of the heart and blood vessels.

But chelation flies in the face of conventional wisdom, which sees cardiovascular disease to result from a build-up of fat or cholesterol in the arteries. Wrong, says chelation. Before the fat build up, the body deposits poisons into the vessel walls that it is unable to eliminate normally, as a kind of 'parking' process. The fat then surrounds this toxic build up, neutralising the poisoning effect on the remainder of the body, and so allowing it to continue functioning normally. Eventually, however, the body can't cope any longer, then clots and blood vessel rupture can occur, leading to heart attacks and strokes. Inflammation has a significant overall place in this disease process.

I had heard of chelation therapy, but only the negative press, so to speak. Kennan's explanation of the treatment, and the disease understanding of its use, was a revelation to me. We had an extended discussion on this and I would advise people with cardiovascular disease to at least look at this alternative prior to or as a complement to any surgery. I also learned that it was successful in a wide range of degenerative diseases, supporting his view that environmentally-caused illness was a problem of epidemic proportions. He now also has cause to see this in action in the Covid crisis.

During this period, Kennan bought a small acreage some miles out of town. It was a wooded retreat on a hill that he then built a family home on. Life was moving on, although he remained single. The town was a suitable adult playground for a single adult professional man, and he was enjoying his medicine again. Ambition seemed out of the window now as he focused on raising his children and developing the property into a retreat called *Ganieda Sanctuary*, which would one day become an extension of his psychospiritual healing interests. But life had other plans.

> The fevers, now some five years absent, came back with a vengeance. I struggled on with practice, being reasonable in the mornings, but collapsed in the afternoons. I maintained good contact with my children, but my health continued to deteriorate and I lost weight rapidly again. Yet, in the back of my mind, I recalled the four-week period it took the illness to spontaneously resolve five years before. But four weeks came … and went.

Then one Friday afternoon when I had taken to bed again, I had a deep feeling, almost a vision: I had gone past the point of no return and would not survive the weekend. Although concerned about this feeling, I did not feel desperate. After deciding it was not time to die, I wondered who to contact and decided on a Scottish radiologist at the hospital, with whom I had a good working relationship. He suggested I come in and that he conduct an investigative process, after routine hospital hours.

I was in the midst of the world of machines that, like hospitals, I had tended to avoid. A scanning process with ultrasound revealed a circular black hole in my liver the size of an orange. When he first saw it on the screen behind me, my overseer remarked:

"Well, I think we've found the cause of the problem!"

I craned my head and saw the hole: "What the hell is that?" I recall enquiring, still feeling calm.

"I don't know" was all the response I received.

Interlude: Kennan had used the analogy of an orange. I metaphorically stopped in my tracks. He had also used it to describe Ann's cancer. I don't think he made the association then or now. Maybe I'll never know. The association of Ann's cancer with an earlier inflammatory breast problem and now Kennan's parasitic illness had not escaped my attention. I had always been of the opinion that inflammation, infection, and cancer have a closer relationship than is currently considered. But I put my musings to one side and let him continue ...

When the radiologist went out of the room I lay back and my mind then went crazy. He had reassured me that it didn't look suspicious, like a cancer, although this did little to settle my emerging nervous state. When he came back, he immediately asked me if he could "stick a needle in it" in his phlegmatic Scottish accent. Anxious to resolve the situation, I agreed.

As the radiologist sucked on the needle, a grey paste steadily filled the syringe. We looked at each other, both realising what this was from the memory trigger given in medical school: Anchovy paste signified an abscess caused in the liver by the parasite amoeba. Common in the West until recent times, it had now all but been forgotten, except for those who had visited Third World countries.

Then all the pieces started to tumble into place, like a jigsaw. I had been to India before Ann died and had a diarrhoea illness when I came back. This in itself was not surprising, but I then remembered after her death, when I was doing the book-burning ritual, I had a very uncomfortable night with a fever and sweating more intense than I had ever experienced before with illnesses like the flu.

So, the diarrhoea was caused by amoeba I had contracted in India. The subsequent illness was when it passed from my bowels into my blood system. Then, a year or two later it settled into the first liver abscess I had with the four-week illness, after we moved south. How was I sure of this? Because now I remembered: Shoulder tip pain is an occasional symptom of liver disease, if the diaphragm is irritated. What I also recognised was that all the episodes had been preceded by stress of one form or another, but on each occasion particularly sudden, surprising, and intense.

But now wasn't the time for analysis – it was time to fix the problem. There was a drug. And I took it in large doses with laboratory monitoring. I was ill for several more days and then I began to feel better, much better, for the first time in many, many weeks. I realised then – as we tend to after the event – how sick I had been. I knew this because during those many weeks I never had a period of respite, and I also realised that what was happening to me had a strangeness about it; it was almost alien.

These two characteristics became an important part of my mental diagnostic kitbag. If, during a period of illness, there is no window of respite, then it is a disease and not caused directly by any immediate stress, something trivial, or minor. Also, if the quality of the affliction does not somehow make sense in the context of the victim's circumstances and their reflection, it is also most probably a disease. The distance between cause and effect can be long and is itself significant.

I recovered. I was followed up later by a specialist who could still isolate amoeba in my bowel, and who further recommended an intense experimental treatment. I declined. I reasoned that the amoeba may be in my bowel, but this is part of the external world and there was no lingering evidence of it being within my body. Many years later, whilst being investigated for other reasons, I asked to have my bowels – or more specifically my faeces – examined again for amoeba. They had now gone. I was not surprised.

Running and maintaining a solo practice at a time like this is difficult. It was one thing that Kennan reviewed in his recovery. He scaled his commitments down somewhat and continued on, whilst asking himself some questions about where he was going professionally. He felt isolated in this regard, although not in his personal life. He had met Ange and settled into a domestic relationship with the white kaftan and a child on the way, when the illness came back – again.

Or so it seemed. Kennan had all the symptoms, but they were just the subjective ones of how he felt and vague pain in his liver region. He didn't have temperatures and did not lose weight. However, the blood testing showed that his body was responding as if the amoeba had returned. He was confused.

Now something strange seemed to possess him, and a feeling that many have experienced at one time or another. One day, as Kennan was driving into work at his practice, he felt overwhelmed with the symptoms and the conviction he could not work. Was this the illness, or was it psychological? He did not know. But he did know he could not work. He simply turned the car around and went home, never to return to his rooms in town.

Kennan was in strange territory. The symptoms generally abated, but some lingered, and lingered. He reduced practice to part-time and worked from home entirely. The stress of running the practice, a small business, and staff was simply too much single-handed. He reluctantly decided to use insurance to cover the financial shortfall, as Ange went into labour and delivered a son. He didn't know where he was going to go from here.

The situation dragged on and on. Kennan was clearly in psychological territory now. He was depressed and confused. Even though there was no objective evidence that the amoeba had returned, his blood tests had showed that he, or more specifically his immune system, was reacting as if it had. At this point the subjective and objective seemed to meet. Somehow his mind, and the memories of the acute illness, had caused his body to react 'as if' he was ill again.

This was a powerful insight that made him question – deeply – his understanding of the relationship between the mind and body. It also made him review so much he had seen in clinical practice and the trivial way that doctors can see illness as being 'all in the mind' or, maybe a bit more scientifically, as psychosomatic. He began to understand how trivial and demeaning this approach was, as well as it having little to say about the relationship between the body and mind and, more importantly, to manage and treat those patients caught between these two stools.

Kennan had his own crisis to deal with. His practice had diminished, his insurance company realised he was vulnerable and tried to get him off the small amount of income insurance he was receiving. Ultimately, he was to challenge them and win, but not without realising how many people suffer the ministrations of such agencies as insurance companies. He realised there were some very dark forces in operation there. Over to him for more …

>My crisis was in a vague and strange hinterland. It lasted years and, in hindsight, I could see it as some kind of dark night of the soul. When I resorted to dreams and my analytic experience, then things began to reveal themselves. I discovered that in Greek mythology Prometheus had a liver problem. It was pecked out each day – devoured – by eagles, as he was staked to a mountain, only for it to recover again each night, for the cycle to continue.
>
>Prometheus was in this torturous position at the whim and will of Zeus, who was the head honcho of the Grecian gods. Prometheus' crime? He had stolen fire from the gods to give to humans as a boon to their existence. Zeus objected to this change in the power-sharing arrangement, so Prometheus was condemned to his punishment through eternity.
>
>Yet all was to end well for Prometheus. How? Well,

Chiron, who was the healer amongst men, chose to change places with Prometheus and become a sacrifice: A seemingly magnanimous act, but one illustrating a deeper wisdom. Chiron was the archetypal healer of mankind. Prometheus brought man consciousness and self-determination, as symbolised by the fire. They had a paradoxical and inverted relationship: Consciousness could suffer at the expense of getting well, or be heightened by being ill.

This was heady stuff, but it made intuitive sense to me. My affliction had been in the liver. It could have been elsewhere, say in my brain, for example. I was drawn to alcohol, which affects the liver, as a way of enhancing psychic or visionary process; that is, consciousness. I was a psychotherapist where it is often necessary to lead clients into trauma, pain and darkness for them to realise where they need to go. Spiritual tradition remembers this; modern medicine has forgotten.

This period of my life was coming to a close with this realization. I knew it simply and unequivocally. My limited practice, now conducted from home, was not financially sustaining. The family would have to make choices about what to do and where to go. I had developed *Ganieda Sanctuary* to a sustainable point, but it would take more, much more, to get it to retreat status. It was then that an invitation came from a strange source and with a surprising outcome.

Ten

I suggested to Kennan that for our next meeting we record the audiotape interview as usual, but use it directly as the relevant chapter in his account, if it went well. I felt we had reached a hiatus, because he was about to take a different turn in his medical career. It seemed a good point for me to recapitulate on where he had arrived at in his journey, by asking what I considered relevant questions. I will simply transcribe the conversation unedited of any significant detail.

"We have arrived at this point without much reference to stories in your practice whilst you were in Albany. Is there any reason for this?"

"I don't think so …" Kennan was a little tentative. "I suppose it is because that whole period was kind of overshadowed by the grief, raising the children, and my own illness. I have some funny stories, but I can't recall anything that altered the way I thought and felt about practice up to this point, or would be instructive to others beyond those I have already given. The main focus, for me, was to take my understanding and experience of mental and emotional issues back into the physical health arena. It was a step toward a genuinely holistic position, I guess.

"If I think about it though, there are a lot of stories; they kind of tumble around inside my mind when I focus on them. I do embed many in my therapeutic work, suitably disguised, of course. They seem more relevant to an educative format and delivery. I can think of plenty I have brought out there, mainly in workshops and retreats in which there is a bit more privacy, containment and respect. Seminars and certainly interviews can be a little too open and might lead to trouble."

"You've experienced trouble here?" I jumped on the lead.

"Yes. I was asked to give a talk one night on alternatives in medical healthcare. I was told it was an invitation-only meeting, although in hindsight it was "deemed open to the public". In the question-and-answer period, I was asked what I thought about AIDS, which was then – some 30-odd years ago – at the forefront of the minds of many.

"I answered candidly. I said that, although there seemed to be a virus involved, this was a long way from saying it was the cause of AIDS. I also pointed out that it was not directly due to sexual promiscuity, but sexual and other practices that weren't being directly considered. My experience of therapy with homosexual men had taught me that the sexual practices of some groups in that community could be quite challenging for normal people to consider."

Interlude: Kennan's views about viruses and their role in disease comes to the fore now we are negotiating Covid. It is of interest to me to see how this unedited piece of writing may reflect and inform his current views about the role of a virus in the pandemic and the way it is being handled.

"I also inferred that the transmission was probably through blood and not sexual fluids in such cases. I also speculated that the virus may not itself be the agent that caused the disease. I added that, during my time in the Osho community, I routinely checked all the devotees who were going to India to see Osho, as it was a requirement of the ashram there. You have to remember that open sexuality and multiple partnerships were often the norm in this community. In that period, I only came across one person who was HIV positive, and he was an intravenous drug user.

"Much of what I said at the meeting is now being openly considered in mainstream, but then it was more heretical. I thought no more about it until I received a phone call from a local reporter asking if I cared to make a response to the letter in the local paper written about me by the then Director of the State Health Department. I was bemused: What letter? And was I referred to directly? No, was his response, but the reporter – along with others – had guessed it was me.

"He sent me the letter. It contained phrases something like: "Of course, a doctor is entitled to his views" and "but sometimes these are frankly dangerous." It went on in that tone. Apparently, a journalist had come uninvited to the meeting and complained. So, I made a carefully crafted response by interview that the journalist printed unedited, as one of my stipulations. I also asked him if he would then contact the Director, who was a medical doctor, and ask if he cared to meet for a discussion. The phone call back from a laughing journalist didn't surprise me: "I asked him, but he refused. He was quite angry and directed this toward you in no uncertain terms!"

"As you may gather, I've been a little more careful since, certainly when I was still in practice. However, now I don't have the concern from the establishment, but I still have a moral obligation to use any stories that I have been privileged to be involved with in a discerning way."

"You won't use them in interviews either?"

"I don't categorise. The stories just come to mind. If there is a public or unfamiliar audience, as in a radio interview, I tend to use them to inform me internally of how to deal with the question before me. If I do use them overtly, they are heavily edited."

"But this is different in workshops?"

"Yes. The boundaries are more private and intimate, and there are agreements or waivers and disclaimers about such material. Personally, I think such formal boundaries like disclaimers are bullshit; I rely on my own moral compass. And, I would like to point out at this time, that with my various conflicts with establishment figures and bodies I have never, ever, had a direct patient complaint – to me, the boards, health departments, or anyone that I know about. If I did, I'm sure I would have heard."

"Fair enough," I responded, "but how has that stance been affected now that you are no longer registered?"

"Well, the confidentiality issues are unchanged. As I said, I have my own moral compass and I respond to that, rather than the dictates of institutional bodies; whom I think suck, by the way."

"Really? But aren't they there to protect the public interest and safety?" My question was a bit tongue-in-cheek, I must admit!

"Of course. But rather like speed cameras, they can serve more than one purpose. Look, I'm sure we'll have more to say about these institutions when you've heard the remainder of my saga. At this point though, with the exception of brushes like the one above, they were not a primary consideration in how I conducted myself."

"So, are you editing what you're recounting to me?" I ventured to ask.

"I wondered when you'd get around to that conclusion! Yes and no. I've changed the client and patient names; that much is easy. I've shifted some of the circumstances around a bit to make them less easily identifiable if I think this is necessary because it is the stories that are important. And they are all true; it is not about protecting the sensibilities of others any more. I take responsibility for my role in all of them and their recounting. I trust the others involved to do the same in their own private world, if not publicly."

I got the point and moved on.

"But there is a wider implication to stories."

We had moved on, definitely, but it was Kennan who initiated the new direction: "The stories to date were more about my emerging views. Of course, these would continue to affect me, as we never stop learning. But they start to take on a different emphasis with experience. If I take chelation therapy as an example, I might explain better?"

"Please do!" I was pleased, as the chelation conversation had resonated strongly with me after our earlier discussion.

"Well, I think I would have administered many thousands of chelation treatments. What is remarkable is that it is so trouble-free. I can recall very few incidents of note and certainly nothing of concern directly related to the treatment itself. What was really impressive was that people got better. Their symptoms diminished and they often avoided prescribed treatments like coronary artery bypass grafts or stents, as well as medication use. That, in itself, is impressive. You'd think, maybe a little naïvely, that the profession would take note, but they don't. Only one trainee general practitioner, a woman, has ever come to see chelation in action, and then only for an hour or so."

"Well, we both know why they do not, so could you expand a little for someone not actively in the health arena?"

"Sure," was Kennan's confident response, "you know there are plenty of what we might call vested interests in medicine. Sometimes these are obvious, like money and prestige, even fame. Others are a bit more psychological, like control and being in the right. Some are even deeper, like not wanting a patient to get better and even keeping them sick. But what really gets up the profession is something that says to them: "Guys, you might have it wrong here!" And chelation certainly does that.

"Chelation says this with its success, which indicates the model we have of cardiovascular disease may be wrong. For the record, in my opinion, it definitely is. It says it by indicating that the field of environmental health and medicine is ignored, when its impact is monumental if chelation is anything to go by. It also says we are wrong by relying on investigations for indications of success, rather than listening to patients' accounts. The first two points are books in themselves, but the last point could be expanded on a bit.

"With chelation, people commonly get symptomatically better. Their angina diminishes or goes away. They can walk for long periods, rather than being restricted to fifty metres. They stop getting dizzy spells … and the list goes on. Then the doctors do investigations and say: "But your arteries are still blocked!" And patients say: "But I feel better!" Then doctors say, "it's the placebo effect," or, "it's all in your mind". Then they dismiss the accounts as being anecdotal and lacking the godlike rubber stamp of so-called evidence-based medicine.

"What the profession is doing here is discounting the patients' accounts, their stories. In effect they are discounting them, not only as patients, but also as people; because our stories ARE us!" Now Kennan was excited. He looked at me with a piercing gaze for several seconds before continuing:

"Maybe, just maybe, the model is wrong. We don't even have to step out of the scientific realm; all we do is provide a different model. What if the old blocked arteries are simply ignored by the body as they make new ones because the others are too damaged? And even if there is a placebo effect, isn't that good? What if all the 'evidence' the profession looks for is restricted to what they think they should measure and ignores other parameters that may be contributing?

"But the issue here is that patients are being ignored. If they say they get better, and this isn't accounted for in the existing way of looking at the problem, wouldn't you be asking why? And then why doesn't the profession ask the same question? Because this is no longer science, it is religion, the religion of dogmatic viewpoints and faith in them. It is scientism, the new religion. We are missing the point: The establishment holds onto its position with religious fervour and, like all good controlling religions, deals with the dissidents unfavourably. I'm being kind here.

"As you may have guessed, or already know, this situation is not confined to chelation therapy. Another example: One thing I heard from the old timers is that they used a paste, known as black salve, to deal with skin ulcers, lumps and bumps – the products of ageing – up to and including skin cancers. They made it themselves and they didn't tell their doctors about it. It is derived from a plant called bloodroot, and compounded into a salve with other readily available agents. Common plants with white sap are also used successfully to treat warts, incidentally, making this something of a principle and art in Folk Medicine.

"In recent years, the press about this has increased, as has the profession's attempt to suppress its use. Although not illegal in itself, there are other methods of control. For example, because it is illegal to make a therapeutic claim without evidence – which, of course, is defined and determined by a controlling body – it can't be advertised or sold as such. My experience with people involved with the manufacture or sale of black salve is that they are hounded with methods that remind me of the Medieval Inquisition and its sale remains illegal in Australia.

"The problem is that there is a mass of anecdotal evidence that it works! But does the profession investigate it? No, because it threatens the existing position and vested interests. But one of the ironies here is that they also use scare tactics, like stories about the damage it does, to frighten people away. Isn't it strange that they should only now use stories when they decry anecdotal evidence elsewhere?

"The argument about evidence is also a circular one, as

chelation practitioners know only too well. To get the required evidence requires the sort of trials and statistical documentation that only well financed institutions like pharmaceutical companies or governments can afford. Are we surprised? But in the meantime, people suffer at the hands of vested interests.

"Medicine specifically, and science generally, is taking on many attributes of religion rather than keeping itself confined to scientific principles, it seems to me. I could go on with other examples, but maybe I've made my point?"

"I think you have," I countered.

"How much do you think Ann's illness and death, and your own brush with it, has influenced your position?" I was keen to return to these issues and explore them further, as it seemed obvious to me that they had a considerable influence on Kennan's views. His answer was to surprise me.

"I think they were already present. Now I am not answerable to the medical profession, I can see that my views are quite inherent and preceded practice, even if I wasn't aware of them at that time. I think what the illnesses taught me – I'm including both Ann and myself here – was an awareness of these views and positions. It kind of brought them to light. In that respect, I am touching on the mystical: Is this karma; were they somehow predestined?"

"Are you saying that you, somehow predictably, had to have the illnesses in your life?" I must have sounded as surprised as I felt emotionally to this statement.

"Let me start with Ann. After she died, I found all her diaries under our bed. One night, armed with a good bottle of red, I sat on the lounge room floor and started reading them. It took me all night and a second bottle of red. I reasoned that she had left them for me to do this, as she could have disposed of them if she had wanted, like I subsequently did with mine.

"It was painful to read her comments about me. It's an experience I would caution, not necessarily against, although it is challenging and can be enlightening. But she also recorded her dreams there and she knew of my interest, both personally and professionally, in dreams and dreamwork."

"What is dreamwork?" I interjected, as my idea of dreams as 'work' was a bit vague.

"Literally 'working with dreams'. Recording them, then adding feelings in and subsequently about the dream – often there's a difference between the two – and then associations, such as a memory, a recent event that seems connected, and so on. Often the dream will kind of reveal itself then, though I discourage using this process for problem-solving in day-to-day reality; I don't think that's the purpose of dreaming.

"It is also essential that we return to a metaphoric and symbolic way of appreciating dream images and dreams themselves. We all have that capacity; it is just that it is a lost art and considered immature relative to our rational and cognitive understanding. I think this is a gross mistake. Rather, I see that such a way of viewing life and the world is a given, a fundamental. If we ignore this, it will operate anyway, and often to our collective detriment."

"A seminar topic?"

"Yes, at the very least. But back to Ann's diaries: What I could see in and understand from her dreams was that a lot of the blame I had taken on myself was actually in the laps of others, most particularly from her childhood and a prior relationship. There were patterns of abuse, often sexual, that surprised me. Whilst it was a disturbing night, the dawn did bring some relief.

"I could also see the matrix from which her illness emerged; not caused, but emerged. This is something I have detected in other young people who develop cancer, and it can wreak psychological havoc on those around and close to them. I came to see that Ann had been pushing me. She wanted me to help kind of sort it out for her but had seduced me into thinking that she was in the adventure as much as I was. Her diaries told me otherwise."

"Seduce is a strong word." I was affected.

"Yes, I didn't think about that too much! It is probably because it was in the sexual arena that these patterns most showed themselves."

"Pray tell ..." I was intrigued, but then added more cautiously, "... but only if you feel that's okay."

"Not sure whether it's okay, but it's time. However, I don't want to merely repeat what we've already discussed. Instead, it would be more helpful to explore the relationship between sex, birth and death. I guess by doing it with respect to her and my illnesses, it may cast a light on where these categories impact in medicine, in both health and disease.

"I believe our society has a good way of protecting us from the full impact of sex, birth, and death. Religion still controls sex with its morality around guilt and shame, but even scientific medicine gets a look in with disease. Medicine gets even more of the share with birth and death, which are now generally conducted in the hospital as some kind of sanctuary and behind closed doors. We don't meet the full emotional and spiritual impact of any of these three processes, which, as you now know, I collectively refer to as the Great Cycle of Existence.

"Not only are they the foundation of our life journey, they are also archetypal and the tools of initiation. This means that they have a powerful initiatory impulse on us, if we are available to their full emotional impact, usually and most effectively in the form of ritual and ceremony. With this comes emotional freedom and hence we obtain a liberation of the soul through being able to navigate according to our own moral position, and not the controlling ethic of others.

"But I'm jumping to conclusions here without outlining how I got there. Up until the point of Ann's illness, my views were a little more extensive and lateral than many, but not really earth-shattering. Certainly, contact with Osho and his community helped explore sexual freedom in a spiritually enlightening and personally liberating way. It also led me to conclusions that caused the significant reflections about the absence of any genuine sexual inquiry in the medical profession.

"By the time Ann was pregnant with Asha, I had pretty much shaken the bonds of my conditioning off and was keen to explore further. I thought and was given the indication that Ann wanted such a path, although in hindsight I suspect she did not. I didn't recognise this at the time, as I've already indicated. Ann was pregnant, so at this point the relationship between sex and birth is fairly clear, and no surprise. But then illness and death added another dimension.

"This was because they all coincided: Ann was pregnant as a result of sex. So far, so good. Then she is found to have a disease close to a birth, becomes ill, and dies within a year. And with the illness her sexuality took on aspects that were liberating, something of a paradox at the time. I also became very libidinous and certainly exploited this to the full after her death. But this exploration was coloured by death, so at the very least there was a devil-may-care attitude to it. Also, people found this, and me, attractive. This was something of a surprise and also a paradox.

"In some ways, I guess I saw that Ann's disease liberated her. Her sexual expression took on a form that I felt to be more her true self. You may be able to read between the lines here, but I don't think further detail is necessary. Even now I see her death as liberating from the torment of her past that she carried, largely unbeknownst to me. Was this torment responsible for her disease? Yes. Did it offer a path of liberation? Yes. Was she prepared to either break through or die? Again, yes.

"Then, more broadly: Is this a function of disease, that it liberates us from the shackles of our conditioning? Does the pattern of the illness itself point to what the specific shackles may be? Are the traumas that appear associated with the disease instinctual, often sexual? How much is sexuality and its lack of development and expression connected to all illnesses and disease? These, and more, emerged in the course of this experience.

"Although I am loath to generalise, I can see what the disease meant for Ann. But this is a long way from saying that the traumas of her conditioning caused her disease. It is also a long way from saying that similar traumas are behind all diseases in a similar way, although there is a grain of truth in this. I believe each and every illness should be looked at individually with no preconditions. In this I respect Jung and see illness, even disease, to be part of the individuation process, or what I would call soul-making.

"This was certainly so with my illness," Kennan continued, almost uninterrupted, "it took all the theories that I had learned in both medicine and analysis, broke them apart during the course of these transitory years, and then reassembled them with experience, insight, and hopefully some wisdom. I had gone on a journey of initiation."

"It was a quite long period of recovery, as you may have gathered." Kennan had begun again. "It was several years. In my outline, in our last discussion, I think I covered the basic pattern of what happened. Here I will try and give you my conclusions in the context of the time, inasmuch as I can. It was also a sustained period when I believed I had an option to leave medical practice but didn't take it. I think that was because, at that time, I didn't feel I had an alternative in my working life.

"I had written a book on medicine in the early stages of my

recovery; it is still around in the filing system somewhere! But I didn't feel that writing was a career alternative until a few years later when an overseas friend and colleague suggested that we co-author a book. This came about in an indirect sort of way and at the end of my recovery. The outcome of this was I believed writing was at best creative and therapeutic, but unlikely as a career. The experience actually led me back to seeing medical practice as my only realistic career option, and hence a move back to the city.

"After the first bout of illness and before the second when the diagnosis finally emerged, I had a strong impulse to explore my heritage. In a practical way, this could have meant going back to England, but instead, I decided to stay in Australia and bought the land that became the retreat; although at this stage it was just a wooded bush block. I think my Jungian background stopped me packing up and returning to England because I realised that the impulse was an inner one about my ancestry and heritage, that I somehow needed to express in this land.

"After the first bout of the parasite illness, and whilst practising medicine and building the retreat, I undertook a training programme with a Druid Order in the UK that could be done by correspondence. I used this as a platform to connect in a more conscious way with my background and heritage. I felt I had left England prematurely in some ways, so I wanted to appreciate it more, and the course provided the platform for me to do this.

"I was able to sustain this process by actively engaging in the building of the retreat, *Ganieda Sanctuary*, including stone circles and other ritual areas. At the same time, I was conducting medical practice where the primary focus was to utilise what I had learnt about psychological medicine generally within the physical setting of malaise, trauma, pain, illness and disease. It was like there were two streams operating, and it may well have been the psychic tension of this that led to the second bout of parasitic illness and ultimately for me to leave practice in the town.

"But I am left with many, many stories. Whilst recovering from the illness these were going through some sort of psychic integration process within me, as I dealt with first my own illness process and second with the recovery. Somehow, I needed to make better sense of what was happening to me … Why else would the illness have revisited me?

"In the recovery period after the second bout, I started writing. This wasn't aimed at any audience in particular, and even publication was not a consideration. I simply needed another way to express what was happening to me. For weeks, even months, I arose early in the morning and wrote for several hours before the household started moving.

"It was at this point that I wondered whether I could return to practice, but return I did, considering at that time that I had little option. As I have explained the insurance situation became just a prolonged exercise in futility that many have experienced. After this was all done and being fairly drained of funds, I tried to integrate practice with my work on developing the retreat. But I was isolated and lacked financial support.

"At this time, I was approached by a businessman who was developing a retreat some three hundred kilometres in a region of the State's southwest. He wanted someone to run programmes there. The problem was … I wanted to stay where I was with what I had already developed! But something had to be done, so after much deliberation, we started a plan around his retreat. This involved developing and driving the educational material that would be delivered, and the place to do that was back in Perth. So, the family packed up and I started general medical practice again, with a view to developing a specific clinic in the city that would support the regional retreat. At least, that was the plan."

"So that didn't happen straightaway?" I asked.

"No, but the process took several years. In that time, I consolidated my views on a more genuinely holistic approach to health and medicine, and was working in a setting, which, to some extent, supported this."

"How would you describe your views at this time?" I asked.

"What I felt I achieved prior to this move was to unify the psychological and physical approaches that were a significant part of my training, qualification, and practice. I had a master's degree in physiological sciences, was a qualified medical doctor and Jungian psychoanalyst, with training in nutritional and environmental medicine. I felt this covered the health spectrum, and I now want to integrate and practice it, not only therapeutically but also educationally. And I felt I had the tools to do this.

"I was, however, aware that my spiritual journey was still running a parallel course. This was awakened with Jung, given substance with Osho, and then further relevance by Druidry with its expression at the home retreat and reinforced by my heritage. I didn't see a place for this and, at that time, it would seem to give the impression to others that it was fringe and new age. This was an appellation I did not want, so I tended to keep that side of my life private. It informed my work, but remained in the shadows.

"This seemed a wise choice, as I kept the prestige and kudos of my profession, without having it threatened in a significant way. And this seemed appropriate as the city and regional project progressed. It wasn't until sometime later that I questioned, revised, and then altered this stance.

"Yet there were some issues that started to become cardinal in my professional approach, irrespective of whether it was the flu, cancer, or madness. I tried to instil a sense of self-responsibility with patients. I dealt with their story and picture of their problem, and I stopped translating or interpreting this into a system or method for my own convenience.

"But, most importantly, I also realised that we had treatment, therapy and healing the wrong way around. Instead of approaching it from the scientific, rational and mechanical perspective, we needed to adopt an orientation that was first and foremost mental or psychological. How to do this I was still learning, and I was yet to give this the name 'soul'."

There was a lot to digest here in Kennan's unedited account; I didn't experience the above section to be immediately transparent. In fact, it confused me somewhat. I suspected there was a mixture of various streams here; including the balance of professional medical and spiritual interests; the considered career alternatives; as well as the vicissitudes of the illness process itself, all of which seemed to be having some sort of governing effect on Kennan and his choices. I allowed things to settle here as they were and move on, trusting the above would become clearer over time.

Eleven

This now seemed a convenient place to pause and have an interlude, which we did, as we both had other commitments to attend to. I also needed to digest the material I had collected to date and begin writing. I hoped this period of reflection might bring some further clarity to the raw data. However, I had a sense that I was in the middle of a larger process and, for the time being, the best I could do was to appreciate where we had arrived at.

In other words, I wanted some temporary order, even relief, before we moved any further; as a consequence, I wrote this short piece, prior to collating all the material that preceded it. There was more to come. I could feel this from the way Kennan was trying to put to bed some of his views from this more historical content and not to leap to where he stood now, some twenty years from this point. And, as I had found some of these conclusions to date challenging, I was sure where we would progress from here would only deepen this whole process.

The first question I addressed was the one of career and this, at least, was beginning to emerge with some degree of clarity. It seemed to me that Kennan's career as a medical practitioner was, in some ways, inadvertent. There was a deeper undercurrent to his choice to study medicine that did not altogether fit well with western medicine. He did not come from a medical background and his practitioner career is dotted with times when alternative pathways seemed to beckon as appealing, appropriate, and more fitted to his nature.

My conclusion was that Kennan's medical practice career was largely the result of personal issues and pressures, rather than the more visionary experience that led to the choice to study medicine in the first place. I suspect, as we progress, that this visionary background may come increasingly to the fore and account for not only his ultimate decision to leave practice, but also to pursue a more archetypally-based medical vocation. However, at this stage, I have only a vague idea about what form this would ultimately take.

Medicine was not in the immediate family structure, farming was. Kennan's father had been drawn to it in a kind of vocational manner and his mother came from a long farming tradition. I surmised that it was health more than illness and disease that interested him. And furthermore, this health interest stemmed from a more community-oriented and cultural basis, even a spiritual one.

Had Kennan not gone to Oxford, then this book may not now be being written. Instead of being immersed in a modern medical framework, it was the 'dreaming spires' of Oxford with its rich history, tradition, and eclectic view of life that enchanted and engrossed him. It was also because he was studying normal health rather than the abnormal variety that so engages modern medicine, which made a difference to him. He was also embedded in an academic and intellectual culture that was itself holistic and multidisciplinary.

Not surprisingly, the choice to stay at Oxford loomed large. The consideration of a potential academic doctorate was on the subject of the neurophysiology of vision that, of itself, may represent his more prophetic tendency. Kennan went to London, largely due to family and career demands, and nearly left within months. His sojourn into the general practice of his youth was a career-saver in this regard, but would it ultimately appeal to his heart? It would appear not, as those days and times of the rural general practitioner, integrated into the social and community structure, are now fast disappearing.

I think the neurophysiology of vision is also a very powerful metaphor for his later attraction to Jung and his imaginative, symbolic approach to both life and personal development. Yet there is something unstated here. The Jung that Kennan dismissed at this time was the one of psychology and its therapeutic application, and not the mature Jung of alchemy, magic and mysticism. Because, it seemed to me, that this was the Jung with whom he had a deeper affinity. With grace, I acknowledge that there are many years yet to unfold, and he may yet return to the mature Jung.

Psychiatry reflected an early option to try and integrate this emerging and continuing vocation, but was thwarted before it ever got off the ground. Kennan was, even at this early stage of the narrative, very dismissive of psychiatry as a medical discipline, let alone a healing one. His career in psychotherapy seemed the logical outcome at the time, yet he retained a continuing attraction to the body that drew him back to general medicine as his basis of practice.

This seems obvious in Kennan's relationship with Ann, where her bodily interests in therapy were a strong feature. However, the very nature of her death made it difficult for him to see this clearly. The return to a more general medical practice career was more the result of the circumstances he found himself in following her death. In a more rural large town, and hence familiar setting, he began an integrative process that saw him emerge as a fundamentally holistic physician, using counselling, education and therapy as his main tools.

Yet this failed to continue: Why? Was it the nature of his own illness? His marriage and new family? Or the desire to have this integrated into a larger psychospiritual picture? It would seem that his own retreat at Ganieda would supply the setting to answer this last question, yet he is drawn away to a venture elsewhere in the Southwest and ultimately to medical practice back in Perth. Again, why?

At that time, Kennan had a business perspective of this decision. He was unable to achieve this goal on his own and needed other input to realise his vision of health based more on setting, or retreat. Yet, at this stage, I am not convinced by this answer. I think he was psychologically running away still, and there were tasks yet unfulfilled, if this were to be realised. What I am convinced of, though, is that the soul orientation and spiritual governing of his life were taking an increased precedence.

What I have deduced from all this is that spiritual governance is the determining feature, although I don't believe Kennan fully realised this at the time. I haven't as yet asked him the question directly, but I suspect the answer would now generally concur with my views.

The reason I say this is because of two trends. The first is that the choices, which seem on the surface to be quite rational and appropriate, seem to directly conflict him at a more – dare I say it – soul level. I am thinking here of his personal and business choices that do not ally with this deeper spiritual trend. It is also why I would have some misgivings, if I were Kennan, about the choice to return to the city under the circumstances described. I also know he both suspected this at the time with his feeling and knows this well now. The second is the pattern of illness, disease and death that has accompanied his journey. Sometimes these are mixed up with the first pattern, at other times they are separate. Yet while the personal choices are more of a psychological nature, pointing to insecurities and fears, the second points elsewhere.

I know little of shamanism, but from my Christian background I do appreciate the metaphor of the Divine Wound, or the wounded healer. I suspect Kennan himself will put his experiences and choices more in this context as we proceed. Yet I am concerned about the amount of suffering he may – will – have to go through before he arrives at the realisation that he, too, is fundamentally a wounded healer, a shaman.

But I am getting ahead of myself and concerned that I am displaying more spiritual and prophetic insights than I believed I had. Is this Kennan's influence, the nature of our relationship, or both? Am I being drawn into my own transformation by interviewing this man?

One matter that Kennan is keen to focus on in our discussions is the client, or patient, so it might be pertinent to outline here a brief and relevant summary of this perspective. These are mainly from Kennan's insights that have been scattered around our talks, which I have edited into some sort of package. I would add that I generally agree with them; any difference would be minor, and in many places they extended on my less appreciable experience and conclusions from my differing perspective.

I have also chosen to place them here because they act as a connection point for the reader with the narrative to date and where it may lead from here. I suspect the fundamentals of Kennan's patient insights won't change as we move into the next part of the story, they will simply mature. This present reflection may also be a reference point for the reader's own experience, providing information and guidance in how to tackle future health challenges, particularly when they involve practitioners and institutions.

Patients (I will be consistent and use this term in this section) want more control than they have at present. This control has a direct relationship to power; because patients often feel powerless in the face of the Healthcare Industry, or henceforth the Medical Industrial Complex (MIC); a term Kennan uses relatively often. And, as Kennan references repeatedly, a sense of personal power is essential to any genuine healing.

But the MIC is not going to relinquish its power. Apart from its relatively tenuous and often insecure positioning, there are simply too many vested interests both with the medical profession itself and beyond, although it would take us too far afield at this juncture to explore them: We are talking here about entities like the various health and medical boards, political interests, and the pharmaceutical industry. Unfortunately, this sense of privilege and entitlement seeps down into the individual practitioner, with rewards of money and social status. But because this sense of power is inflated, limited and in many ways not authentic, there is a dynamic of trying to retain it … at the expense of others – the most susceptible being the patient.

Unless the patient develops their own sense of power – because they won't get it from the practitioner, profession or the MIC – then they will readily lose control of what is, essentially, their own illness and disease. This power comes from within, born of experience and qualified with information. In Kennan's terms, stand up to your doctor; if he or she can't take it, they are not right for you. If they can, you have the foundation of a cooperative and creative relationship, and one that is additionally a foundation of healing.

This demands self-responsibility. The shadow patterns of fear, guilt and blame have little if any place if genuine healing is your intention, otherwise they simply engender a false sense of power and control in the practitioner, and are anathema to healing. And self-responsibility is not limited to medicine, of course. It demands the ability to own and deal with your own shadow; being your fears, desires and any psychological games. All those things that help develop a sense of self, but often a pseudo or false one. A genuine sense of self that owns all its thoughts, feelings and behaviours is a necessary pre-requisite to genuine self-responsibility.

As Kennan points out, this is all easier said than done. He sees seminars and workshops for this understanding as being important; where these patterns can be explored with stories, examples and role-playing. It is something the family can engender. I know that both Kennan and I take this task seriously with our children, although none of whom are in the health professions. I wonder why?

It is very difficult to form any sort of relationship that includes dialogue with the MIC; even those of us within the profession have great difficulty. But it is possible to develop one with your practitioner. Pointers include: Unless you feel heard; unless there is some sort of genuine emotional contact; unless the practitioner is willing to share something of themselves ... then, forget it and move elsewhere.

Your practitioner must be connected to their own healing process, which includes their own wounding and trauma, to help you connect with yours. Because unless you can or are helped to make such a connection, then the best any problem will get you is a band-aid; that is, symptomatic relief but not a genuine cure, which relates to healing. Your practitioner should encourage and support you on your own journey, and not foist their protocol on you if it is incompatible, inappropriate for you or otherwise unacceptable to your belief system.

Your practitioner should also accept any differences in the way you model and approach your health. This puts the demand back on the patient to explore alternatives and other possibilities. Both people in this exchange need to be open-minded, so the discussion can become a genuine sharing and a dialogue. Both of you need to appreciate the emotional, mental and spiritual realms if healing is your path.

It is worth remembering that most patients go to a doctor

because they are concerned, even frightened. This simple fact should never, never be taken advantage of.

Twelve

"It's been a while, hasn't it, Kennan?"

"It has, Ian, it has."

We were quite familiar with each other now, both of us knowing we had forged a friendship that would sustain beyond this project. In fact, it was the blossoming friendship that threatened the continuation of this work, in some ways. This was because I was beginning to appreciate and understand Kennan beyond the way I had originally surmised. But it was also because the friendship itself may sabotage the project, by not giving it the creative edge it might need to continue.

I now think that the preceding chapter may go some way to explaining this, but it also meant a change for me. I now felt more on an equal footing with Kennan, when previously I had looked up to him. Maybe I had absorbed some of his 'patient advice' as well? This change allowed me to draw some conclusions that I never would have prior to knowing him this well.

We discussed this, of course. Kennan likened these dynamics to the creative challenges that a therapeutic relationship can go through, and I could see this. The change in the relationship dynamic – specifically the power dynamic – could have ended the project, but not necessarily the friendship, into which it could have changed. But it didn't. Why not?

I think it extends from what I was expressing in the preceding section, where I was trying to differentiate the interpersonal from the transpersonal or spiritual issues. The same could be true here, in that we both recognised a larger purpose to our relationship, and were prepared to relatively sacrifice the immediate ongoing personal relationship in favour of this.

Was I just realising this, maybe as a result of the preceding reflections? Did Kennan know this all along and let me make the choice? I did not then and still don't know. All I know is that he then rocked my temporary equilibrium and changed the flow into risky territory.

"I wonder what would have happened if our friendship had a sexual potential?"

"Jeez, Kennan! What the hell do you mean by that?"

"Well, we've kind of progressed through a creative transition in our relationship. As things stand professionally at the moment, should sex emerge therapeutically in such a relationship, the choices are that you either put it in other more objective terms like 'transference', or you finish the therapy and fuck!"

The man knew how to throw me.

Then he followed up with: "What we don't currently do is properly integrate the sexuality into the therapeutic relationship and then use it as a catalyst to or for something else in a creative or spiritual sense."

And that tipped me over the edge mentally! "OK, you've got me there. I'll need to reflect on this. Maybe later?"

"Sure, I'm confident we'll come back to it. Want to go somewhere else? I was struck by the comment recently about the paucity of stories from my practice days in the Albany practice, so I've come up with a couple. Neither of them seems mind-blowing at present, but they do seem to have something in them about territory we might move on to. Want to hear them?"

"Sure."

"The first was an eighty-year-old man who came to see me for a repeat script. He accepted one of his medications, but asked me whether he needed to continue on the one for his blood pressure. I asked him why he questioned this one. He told me that, at eighty, there was little to look forward to, but – and he made a tense fist – this is one of them. I had the wherewithal to realise he was talking about sex and not clouting someone!"

Following the laughter, I asked him what he did with the request.

"Took him off that med, as I reasoned they were giving him the erectile dysfunction he was hinting at."

"Did it work?"

"Well, I did get a phone call from his wife a couple of weeks later, asking me if I'd changed his medication. I said I had adjusted them a bit. She asked me to return to the original regimen as, in her words; "he was very well controlled before you changed them"! I'm sure we'll cover the issues here, sex and medications, though not necessarily together." He sipped his coffee with a smile.

"The second story is about a young woman who had been diagnosed with schizophrenia. I only ever saw her once professionally, but was hounded by paranoid phone calls subsequently for a period, before they abruptly ceased.

"Then, many months later, I awoke early one morning and wondered what had happened to her. Had her delusions changed? Was I no longer the paranoid subject of them? Then the phone rang: It was her. She was ringing from Sydney to tell me – angrily – to stop having her followed, definite I had organised the 'surveillance'!

"Like the first, funny, but with something else in it. She had called me from thousands of miles away at the very time I was thinking about her and for the first time in ages. Had she picked up on me, or vice versa? Who was the mad one? And what about the telepathic implications?"

Maybe the third brush with quantum physics or psychic

territory, following the two around Ann's death? Time to move on, but like the first story, I was sure we'd return to what was contained in it.

There was an air of desperation about the return to Perth; I felt it in the telling, and even Kennan acknowledged he knew this at the time. He had developed his rural home at Ganieda to a point that it could be used as a retreat, but there was a lot of work that needed to be done. But it wasn't the work that was the problem; it was the finance, or lack of it. Now Kennan had recovered from his illness he was doing some practice from home, but it and he were now too far away from mainstream to be able to provide the necessary income to maintain and develop the retreat project there.

The offer from the businessman in the Southwest seemed substantial. Their aims were common and they had joint interests that could merge; he had the developed location – which Kennan did not have as yet – and Kennan had the required expertise. Much planning then ensued and further necessary building started. Yet the project demanded a move to Perth, as there needed to be a presence in there to support the retreat, and the asset of the medical persona was a vital part of the business mix.

Kennan regretted leaving Albany and what remained of his practice post-illness, but he felt it was in the best interests of the family to move to Perth again, as well as developing his own professional interests further; not only with respect to this retreat project, but also with like-minded personnel there. So, he buried his concerns, including those that surrounded the family business set-up of the Southwest retreat, and made the move. His home and partially developed retreat there would go into mothballs from the development perspective and continue as a personal retreat only, as the family became increasingly ensconced in city life.

This didn't sound good, even as I recorded the conversation. It seemed to me that there was not only some desperation, but also some questionable assumptions being made. I think Kennan had a vision of a supervening position that contained all his interests, but it seemed ungrounded, abstract and too expansive. It sounded like, and could well be another instance of, his spiritual ambition not being in harmony with his personal circumstances.

Yet things were to develop with promise. After finding a suitable practice at Point Walter Medical Centre to start working from, Kennan then developed a relationship with the managing director. Point Walter was one of many that constituted the national corporate group. As Kennan continued to build his practice, this caught the Director's eye. He was also impressed about Kennan's ideas for a clinic model of a holistically integrated nature, seeing this as a more community-based model than the way general practice was developing at that time.

The Director further understood that although this clinic model was for Kennan a basis for his interest in education and retreats, there was the possibility of using the model across the range of corporate medical centres in the group's possession. Being the largest of its kind in Australia, the promise was good indeed. The move to the city now seemed well-founded. As Kennan continued in the general practice part of the building, the new HealthQuest Clinic was being fitted-out in another section. It was equipped with room to provide seminars and other educational and group delivery formats to complement his practice interests.

With the ensuing optimism, Kennan and Ange bought a house nearby and settled into city life. There was an increasing sense that the whole platform was becoming less dispersed and more integrated. Kennan developed other professional relationships, as well as a network around his ideas and their development. He was most particularly gratified that the educational component was gaining momentum.

But how did Kennan find returning to routine general practice, even though this promised to be a short-term move?

What surprised him most was how little had changed at the coalface of practice. There were new drugs, but not any of a significantly different class from when he first qualified. In many ways, it was like 'getting back on the bike'. He was able to keep his more complementary medical ideas away from the general practice itself, as the new clinic started to function and his more holistic approach appealed to his growing practice and, to a lesser extent, some of the other practitioners.

The biggest thing that Kennan had to come to terms with was corporate medical practice. This was something he had not experienced before. He initially found it difficult to have his mode of practice somewhat dictated to by the corporate administration. Even though it was generally a cooperative relationship, the loss of autonomy and the power to change things in response to practice needs was now foregone.

There were other concerns: the influence and extent of involvement of other agencies in practice itself were appreciably greater than before. The centre itself was run by a company where shareholders were now part of the mix. And the biggest shareholder of this company was a major pathology group. Kennan found this relationship a little unhealthy, but reasoned that it did not influence his choice of pathology referral or its extent; that is, in a direct manner. Indirectly things were somewhat different.

There was, and still is, little subtlety about the influence of the pharmaceutical industry. Apart from the perks, they were responsible for a significant amount of the further education that practitioners were now compelled to undergo to maintain their professional status and hence standard of living. The value of this education Kennan found to be generally poor and motivated by other rather obvious business interests. What was more concerning was that this provided much of the 'evidence' for evidenced-based medicine and hence the protocols that practitioners were and are increasingly expected to conform to.

Kennan was also deeply concerned about the association of the pharmaceutical industry with the Therapeutic Goods Administration, not only in pharmaceutical regulation but also in dictating to other more natural therapeutic approaches. This concern was only to grow over time, he pointed out, to his current position of advocating freedom of alternatives to the individual in all aspects of their health; be it from herbal alternatives, but also embracing choices in wider issues like vaccination and euthanasia.

It was not hard to see the public perception that there was, and is, too much influence from the pharmaceutical industry. In fact, what concerned Kennan now was that pharmacy was seen as an essential component of general practice, with little in the way of alternatives. He also became concerned about the extent of pharmaceutical usage and the arguments that were used to back it – issues like medical statistics, evidence-based medicine and the like seemed to be used not necessarily with the intent they were originally developed for.

There was the institutionalisation of medicine itself. The legal influence was now rife and, in a somewhat sweeping opinion, Kennan came to see that legal concerns had become the major influence in the practitioner's choice of management. Although legal interference was relatively uncommon, it hung around a practice and the practitioner's choices in health delivery like a bad odour.

Then there was – is – the actual control of practitioners themselves. It seemed to Kennan that the various boards that dictated what was perceived to be good practice or otherwise were often poorly equipped to do this properly, and seemed to serve more political gods, his own prior and later experience notwithstanding. The number of practising practitioners on such boards is usually low and often it is lawyers who dictate terms. Of course, public welfare is paramount, but to him it seemed that this became a mantra to be brought out if censure were demanded and to excuse punitive actions.

For Kennan, this brief overview was enough. When he read this short section subsequently, Kennan was to remark that there was enough material to "write a book" on each of these topics alone. Many have done this, but he was also keen in our discussions that these issues were to be put into context. He saw it as being disempowering and uncreative to engage in these arguments beyond a point. He was keener to seek alternatives and answers to the problems posed. In effect, he believed that the medical profession itself was in need of healing and to do this, as with the individual, it had to come from self-management.

In summary: Kennan found these difficulties oppressive and stressful to deal with. He noticed that most practitioners ignored their psychological effect and hence their personal impact, whilst at the same time operating according to the dictates of the various institutions that sought to regulate and control medicine, which were not usually in the practitioners' best interests. His approach was to understand how they operate and see if he could pursue his professional interests with as little interference as possible; in other words, he decided to 'fly under the radar'.

What about practice itself: how did Kennan's experience of these changes affect his modus operandi?

Firstly, he referred back to the discussion, immediately above, indicating that practice itself has to be understood in this wider sphere of influence and control. What he decided to do was to render unto Caesar what was Caesar's; in other words, while he offered a general practice service whilst developing the HealthQuest clinic, he would do this accepting the professional guidelines that governed it. The addendum was that behind the closed doors of his consulting room, he could bring in the latitude and alternatives that his experience had to offer.

Over a short period of time, Kennan had developed a practice following, which rapidly shaped itself around patients who were looking for more than prescriptive answers and were concerned about their health in a way the various governing institutions were not responding to or addressing. As the new clinic took shape, he was then able to offer these alternatives in practice for those who chose them. As there was a clear distinction between his general practitioner services and HealthQuest, tacitly respected by the other practitioners, he was able to operate in this way, until other events supervened.

But if I focus on what it was that Kennan brought to general practice, it seems to me that there are several ways in which to explore this. I have managed to pare these down to four, although they do tend to overlap. The first is the health model that is being offered by the practitioner. He had trained as a modern western medical doctor and practised as such. This approach took in two broad considerations: the manner in which he was trained, and the different influences he has been exposed to and integrated into practice through his life experience.

Kennan was most concerned about the loss of practice as an art and the increasingly and exclusively scientific approach. This translated to less focus on the patient's story, but also the physical examination, and then the reliance on investigations that were predominantly of a pathological orientation. Not only this, but also patients had been taught in various ways to see parameters like blood test results as reflective of their health and choices in any management.

What this amounts to, in Kennan's opinion, is a distancing of the health focus from the actual physical body of the patient and then giving a distorted mental picture. This leads to a loss of a connection of a symptom with a problem in the patient's mind. It amounts to a loss of personal management and self-determination in matters of health.

This is also not helped by the practitioner, both often eschewing a proper physical examination and also not engaging in an educational role with the patient. The latter could be seen as the practitioner wanting to keep power and control, although it is actually more complex than this. The practitioner is simply not taught to educate, and he or she is increasingly trained in practice by people who are not clinicians. Education in symptomatology prior to the employment of investigations Kennan saw as an important role, which demands clinicians as well.

Kennan's life experience, and how much he brought to the consultation process, had been a matter that vexed him to this point in time. Whilst his experience in non-medical fields has definitely broadened and deepened his approach, there was a limit to how much he could or was allowed to openly express this. So, a lot was done covertly, but this dichotomy amounted to a psychic division and was appreciable, as I have already outlined. It could and would only increase over time.

This perspective inevitably flowed into what Kennan saw as the reinstatement of the importance and centrality of the doctor-patient relationship. This was the second point, in my opinion, even though it overlapped the first. Obviously, when a more teaching orientation is within the health model employed, there is a greater emphasis on this relationship. There is an increasing tendency for this to be diminished in favour of a more rational, scientific and objective approach driven by protocols. That this is failing a confused and fearful public is all too obvious.

In Kennan's mind, this is what tradition has to offer. There is something that can happen in the therapeutic relationship that can be healing in and of itself. That this brings in intimacy, and hence emotional connection and the thorny issue of sexuality on occasion, and is why it is negated and denied, when instead it should be engaged and appreciated. Yet it points to something magical that disciplines like hypnosis and the art of suggestion hint at. His experience in analysis and psychotherapy had given him the tools to utilise the relationship dynamics, but he saw that mainstream was a long way from accepting them, and for reasons he found spurious and self-serving beyond patient welfare.

The third area of concern is often so ignored it is not seen. Kennan refers to this as the 'setting'; that is, where the consultation process is conducted. Commonly in the modern era, this is in a sterile, clinical and uncreative environment, which is divorced socially and psychologically from the patient's daily life. It does not give the practitioner wider reference points in health management, such as seeing the patient in the home setting. There is also a tendency to ignore other things that may have a role in health and healing. What about artwork instead of pharmaceutical or branded models of dissected hearts or kidneys? Where is the role and influence of nature, particularly domestic animals?

The setting is also now dominated by the computer screen. The arguments for this are overwhelming and seemingly persuasive, although this is in response to a flawed model, in Kennan's opinion. The computer screen now dominates the relationship and beyond. The patient becomes a statistic for comparison to protocols and subsequently management. Also, the screen detaches the practitioner from engaging with the patient and allows them both to deny the emotional dimension.

Yet this fourth dimension, the emotional or spiritual component, is huge in Kennan's view. From his experience in depth psychotherapy, Jung in particular, emotion is the vehicle of and to the soul. And isn't it the suffering of the soul that seeks out a doctor? We are troubled by what we feel – our doubts, fears and insecurities – as much or as well as our physical symptoms that themselves may be the emotions crying out. Now, because science has become divorced from art, and spirituality from the mechanics of the body, we have lost contact with these greater, wider, deeper and mysterious dimensions that have an imperious and even determining role in our health; or so Kennan believes.

Such were the influences that Kennan brought to the table but hoped to see a more open flowering of them in the developing new clinic. But he was to receive a savage blow.

The Director of the corporation had resigned. He was not a doctor, but he did have a visionary view of the direction of healthcare; why else would he have supported Kennan with the development of the clinic? His resignation was essentially a response of the board to concerns about his business and financial direction, including such ventures as Kennan's new clinic. Unlike the retiring Director, and like the medical profession, the board seemed short-sighted to the larger picture, probably for pecuniary reasons.

At the meeting with the new Director, Kennan and his colleagues realised the writing was on the wall for their project. The new Director was a clever medical doctor who saw the future of the company along party and governmental lines. This came at the same time that the Southwest business partnership started to founder, mainly because of the family nature of the business, which initially Kennan had concerns about. Kennan threw in the towel.

He decided to consolidate, and relocated the HealthQuest

clinic elsewhere in the complex and in association with the pharmacy there, following an invitation from the pharmacy's owner, Thomas. This particular pharmacy provided a lot of support to alternative practitioners and their pharmaceutical needs as a compounding pharmacy. The association with the pharmacy owner was sound and to a common interest. Although very much a scaled-down model of what had been originally conceived, and now minus the education component, it was more manageable. It was also a necessary readjustment with the gradual diminishing and ultimately loss of the Southwest arm of the project, which was the reason he had come to the city in the first place.

Oh, how the dice falls!

For a few years, Kennan maintained this balance of further developing the HealthQuest Clinic with Thomas and his now flourishing general practice within the same building. His intention was to gradually translate his professional profile into HealthQuest as it matured and developed, and to scale down his GP profile, so as not to let his patients down. The factor that was missing from this was the original one that had brought him to the city in the first place: the retreat project.

As the new clinic became populated with doctors and a psychologist, the original vision became diluted with the practicalities of maintaining a focus within mainstream medicine. In Kennan's view, the clinic started to resemble a mainstream practice with the only essential difference being the offering of natural approaches to healthcare, rather than a primary emphasis on pharmaceutical medicine. The mode of practice of the doctors there was effectively the same as mainstream, along with fears of the supervening administrative and other institutional bodies whose excessive presence in medicine most concerned him.

Albany and the fledgling retreat of Ganieda was also

beckoning. He had been away too long. Kennan made a decision, or more a raft of decisions. He decided to entirely cede his involvement with the clinic to Thomas. He felt it had probably gone as far as it could go in the development of the concept, being the first to gather a number of holistically-inclined medical practitioners into one practice. He would maintain a presence there as a practitioner and would give up his general practice entirely.

Kennan decided that maybe it wasn't in practice that he would have an impact and leave any kind of legacy; although the HealthQuest Clinic he started still operates successfully to this day. He decided it was time to write again, even in spite of his earlier experience. His creativity was stirring, as was his longing for home. The family sold their home in the city and returned to country, where he wrote one week and then commuted to the city for medical practice in the clinic for the next, in a fortnightly cycle that was to last about three years.

I asked Kennan what had led to the decision to write.

"I first wrote after the last episode of the parasite illness. As I explained, it was in a handwritten hardcopy, as this was many years before. But I do believe it had a profound effect on recovering and finally healing from the illness, which is interesting in itself.

"Then, several years later we hosted an international Druid conference at home. After this, the Chief of the Druid organisation, a writer and psychologist, wrote to me convinced I was an alchemist of old and was using the home retreat to explore and make the so-called elixir of life, the mythical entity of longevity and eternal youth! Although he was somewhat tongue in cheek with his assessment, he did point to my interests in health being about rejuvenation and longevity. And this made sense; in his own way, he identified the spiritual core at the heart of my medical career.

"So, we set about writing a book about all this, but it didn't work for us as a co-writing project. We were individuals and creative ones at that, but the team approach didn't gel. So, after I had done the outline and written the bulk of the book in my own inimitable style, it was confined to a neighbouring drawer to my earlier effort. I decided, with his criticisms of my approach, that I was not a writer. At this stage, I had met my future colleague from the Southwest retreat and decided to pursue that avenue.

"When I ceded my interests in HealthQuest, apart from remaining as a one-week-in-two part-time practitioner, it was because the creative urge had arisen strongly in me. I should point out that creativity had been part of my early life; I used to win art prizes at school. I think what this move demonstrated is that true creativity can take many and varied forms, simultaneously and over time. As a psychotherapist, I realised I was a storyteller, a wordsmith. I wanted to find out if writing was an extension of this in spite of my earlier misgivings."

I interjected: "So you believed, at that time, that the route of medical practice was not your fate or contribution to the world?"

"Well, I had cause to give it serious question, hadn't I! But seriously, I wanted to take stock. I was then approaching sixty and felt that a new stage in my life and maybe a fresh direction was opening up for me. I needed to pursue this. It may not have been entirely fair on the family, but I owed it to myself, I thought."

I was left to ponder the role of creativity in health and healing as Kennan then discussed his writing. Practice considerations had been put on the back burner during this period, except as a means to put food on the table, although continuing to provide insights to him and alternatives to patients so looking.

I was drawn to discussing Kennan's writing further. He had written, not only about medicine, but also a personal memoir, and a fictional work with sexual and supernatural overtones. It seemed that he did this as some sort of creative respite in the time away from commuting to and working in Perth; another psychic divide seemed apparent to me.

Personally, I feel not to do this when I write in these areas. I believe that we are being prematurely drawn into speculative views and conclusions about the state of health and medicine; so, was Kennan doing this too? It seemed to me that the pattern in his writing was pointing in another direction; simplistically away from medicine to a memoir (of sorts), and then into areas of sexuality and spirituality. Another path was beckoning – one that finally placed him within the psychospiritual stream that so informed his life. But he was – temporarily – to eschew this.

Kennan was now at another juncture. Although he would have retired entirely from medical practice at this point, could he afford to do so? He still had family duties and the education of his and Ange's son, Tristan, to deal with. Practice at the clinic was sustaining him, but the travel was becoming a chore. He had not been able to resurrect sufficient practice in his home town whilst writing every other week to stay in the rural region exclusively.

Then he received an attractive offer from a large mainstream private and non-corporate practice close to Perth, in Mandurah, through one of the more enlightened doctors there, to look at a mind-body medicine clinic model like the originally conceived one with Thomas at HealthQuest, but this time with more apparent practitioner support.

Although at one level this seemed a revisitation of old ground, Kennan felt that only such a challenge may sustain him in practice, at least until his son's schooling was complete. It portrayed a scope that the HealthQuest Clinic as he had conceived it could not achieve, and may yet be the link to his educational and retreat dreams. Or so he surmised.

Thirteen

The family were on the move again; this time to Mandurah, a city to the south of Perth. I was now appreciating the chronology; from the early days when Kennan's account flitted back and forth in time, there now appeared to be a more regular and linear sequence. But I was also concerned that, educational aspects notwithstanding, the account was becoming more of a memoir and losing some of more edgy and controversial aspects – and the last thing we both wanted was for this account to be another doctor's self-indulgent and even narcissistic account of righting the wrongs of the medical profession.

Had things gone differently with the original HealthQuest Clinic project and its alignment with his home retreat in the south near Albany, Kennan reasoned that he could have worked from this combined platform, as his ambition would have been fulfilled; or, at the very least, finally headed in the right direction. However, at this point in time this was not be, and he also had his son's education to consider.

The approach from a large general practice in Mandurah seemed promising. He had formed an alliance with one of the doctors who practised there, who was also a partner in the medical centre business. For Kennan, this meant that the medical corporation was internal; that the partners ran the centre business, and were not also a management board beholding to external shareholders.

The partner, James, came from a similar British background to Kennan and had gravitated to medicine via the arts at university. He also had the distinguishing feature of social justice at the health delivery level, which Kennan now recognised as a relative necessity in his professional associations. James also had experience in mental health, youth and addiction medicine. Effectively, he ticked all the boxes as a potential colleague.

What Kennan and James concocted to do was to develop an arm to the medical centre that dealt with mind-body medicine and holistic health; effectively, the original concept of HealthQuest in all but name. In that way, it was more like the original concept in the earlier corporate practice, where Kennan had envisioned the project integrated within modern medicine and general practice more generally, incorporating health education, and not simply as the niche practice it had become with Thomas. This time, he felt he had more medically-based support.

What clinched the move was the needs of the family. There was suitable schooling there for his son that Albany could not provide, and the deteriorating health of one of his wife's parents in Perth cemented the choice. The retreat project was to be put on hold once again, although this time his wife wanted to remain close to the city, so the moth-balled future development of the retreat was now in his hands and no longer contingent upon the family's needs into the future.

As I knew the ultimate outcome of this choice, I was not as uneasy as I would have been if Kennan were presenting it to me as a current option. It seemed to me that the pattern of the disparity of his vision and the personal elements to the choice was repeating itself. I would have counselled him not to make this move, but one of the differences between he and I was that Kennan would back his feeling in a way I would not. I would have played it differently; maybe safer, but differently.

One reason I felt this way was because of a discussion we'd had about his role in the city corporate general practice. When he started again as a general practitioner he had thought: "If I were to ever start up a practice again, I could end up an alcoholic, deregistered, or dead." He told me this is what he had reflected at the time, because of the demands of starting a practice from scratch. This seemed to me a strangely prophetic utterance.

Was Kennan simply challenging the fates or being prophetic? Didn't he know the risks he was taking? His alcohol intake, generally higher than the commonly recognised normal or healthy, was unproblematic when he was writing, but rose again with the move to Mandurah. It was once again being used to deal with the emotional stresses of starting a practice, rather than an intake simply undertaken in the social context. He told me that the occasional binge, which he sometimes used rather like a psychedelic experience to access altered states of consciousness, became difficult to contain. There were distinct features of using alcohol to escape, in the psychological sense; but to escape where? He still had not found home.

To this point of time, however, alcohol had never been a concerning feature of Kennan's daily working life, although it had been close on occasion. He still prided himself in not using pharmaceutical drugs such as sedatives, believing alcohol was known and safer in his down time. I was concerned about this argument and would have challenged him should it have been a current issue. Yet he did not avoid being open about this feature of his life, and I knew that he had engaged professionals for feedback, comment and advice at several points in his career.

At the same time, the Ganieda retreat was to undergo a development in Kennan's absence. The property had been approved for subdivision as a designated health retreat for several years, and now he and his residential caretaker had the wherewithal to enact this. He would like to have been more involved in this process and was sad about this, but left it in the caretaker's seemingly reliable hands.

At this point I was compelled to ask myself: What did and do

I make of this man? I liked Kennan; he was affable, and could be charming, although there was a distinct touch of the devil about him. I felt that whether I liked him or not was something he was not trying to determine or impress upon me. Was he a slow burning genius, or simply an alcoholic in the making? If I lapsed into my training, he might be classified as narcissistic – a conclusion I had come to before – but it was a deep kind of narcissism, self-serving in a way that didn't clearly identify the self that was being served.

There were tinges of Faust in the contracts Kennan made with others, and himself. But I inclined to the view that he served his creative 'daimon', and that it was this that dictated his choices and direction. Certainly, he is intelligent and very knowledgeable, but the genius that the word daimon implies could be a bit far-fetched. I prefer to see daimon to indicate a person's passion, innate skills and destiny, and I am sure he would concur. Maybe his own picture will only be determined in hindsight, when the story is over and what is bequeathed in any legacy can be seen and appreciated in this light.

I don't think Kennan himself understands what drives him. Some think him crazy, although he has never doubted his sanity. He has a deep trust that 'the gods' – his words – determine his fate and that his job is to pursue what is ordained for him to undertake. And what does he see that as being, I would ask him?

"To change the direction and face of medicine," I'm sure would be his prophetic reply, I imagined.

"You, yourself?"

"I know I am not alone, but I am compelled to be part of any future change," he may go on to explain. "Because it must change; yet it will only creatively change if this is done by those who see its flaws, darkness, and sometimes obviously evil ways. If I am a part of that process and help define what it is changing to, then I have done my job."

"Even though it would drive you mad, make you alcoholic, or even kill you?" I would continue.

"Yes. I have a sense of the deep pattern, buried in tradition, to which medicine and healing must return. Because of and in this I have a responsibility, but exactly what my role would be beyond this point does not seem mine to determine."

I decided to cease this hypothetical conversation, as I trusted it would emerge and clarify in where the account went from this point. I was also more than a little nervous undertaking it, as I didn't know where it might lead me, or did I? I didn't know whether I was ready for that, as yet. Just yet.

I don't think it is necessary to recount the story of his last years in medical practice in any great detail, except as some sort of postscript, or metaphoric epitaph. Ultimately Kennan chose a metaphoric rather than literal death. I did fleetingly wonder if he would have chosen a literal one, were it to suit his deeper ambition, but he saw that this would have been a failure, an unnecessary martyrdom; one that too many of his colleagues have, and do, unwittingly choose.

There were no particular signs of what the next three years would bring when he first went to Mandurah. Kennan was buoyed by James's enthusiasm and position of influence and control in the practice, and by the initial support of some of the other practitioners. The doctors were a varied multicultural crew of predominantly British extraction, with an increasing number of overseas and particularly South African members.

The partners of the centre were formed from a small group of the practitioners. They owned and controlled the centre and its direction, and seemed a reasonable lot, also – initially – he did not seem to pose any sort of threat. However, this was largely out of ignorance on their part of the role he would take there over time. Additionally, the staff seemed friendly and worked well as a team, supported by a practice manager who did not wield a significant stick of any kind.

Kennan settled into a rhythm and started building a practice, yet again. He wasn't listening to his own story, it seemed. Whilst his involvement at the HealthQuest in Perth tapered down in response to the development at the Mandurah centre, he started to consolidate his approach to what he saw as genuine holistic medicine within the current medical environment, with a potentially more expansive future than the clinic as it had become after he had ceded ownership and responsibility of HealthQuest.

The broader coastal city community supported him and he began to become a hub of kinds, assisted by James and a psychologist in the practice. However, if ever he took his views into the broader forum of case presentations to all the practitioners, he began to sense threat, even jealousy.

This was reinforced by the centre being a hub of another kind: the training of doctors as specialists in general practice. He felt his views were seen as being potentially disruptive and iconoclastic to those involved in the training, and hence unwelcome. This was a dynamic or pattern of a different kind, and one that Kennan quickly decided to avoid. He took no further part in the case presentations or training sessions. Instead, he started to run his own educational seminars for the general public away from the centre.

Kennan actively developed and supported his developing practice, although was concerned about some of the wider community and social features. These included distant workplaces (the 'fly in–fly out' phenomenon) causing family disruptions, the prevalence of drugs of addiction and addiction-related problems particularly as this overlapped his interest in mental health, as well as the amount of domestic violence in the broader community.

This caused a contraction of a different kind. It meant that his outreach to the community became limited, as Kennan charged only private rates: he believed everyone should contribute to their own healthcare. He routinely did not take on mental health problems where drug addiction was a dominant feature; there was James for this. In fact, he began to see the wider social dimension of mental health disturbances more generally. He began to question his previously held and now tenuous position of seeing mental healthcare as a legitimate component of modern medical practice; a view that was to gain a wider perspective and conviction when he left practice.

Yet even with these emerging and concerning features Kennan continued. This was in spite of his own health undergoing a scare, when he developed chest pain and was hospitalised with what was diagnosed as pancreatitis. He was reassured his heart was okay, and he came to realise that the pancreatitis was an incorrect diagnosis. It was based on a blood test only and assumed to be alcohol-related. That it followed alcohol input was of no doubt, but it was an assumption; it was a reaction to the codeine that was in the analgesia he took for the resultant headache. Normally he used paracetamol only for such occasions. On this occasion, this combined preparation of paracetamol and codeine was all that was in the house that night. This has been further confirmed by having no subsequent episodes – and avoiding codeine, of course. Another misdiagnosis, he felt, and again at the social level.

Kennan returned to work and saw some significant changes occurring around him. The manager had resigned and was replaced by one from a pharmaceutical industry background. Her brief was to 'rebrand' the practice and centre to meet the social changes that were occurring in and impacting on private medicine, which had led to a reduction in patients, as cheaper more convenient medical services were sought elsewhere in the city. She also brought an efficiency that was based on time-based services directed toward financial return.

Obviously, this did not suit what James and Kennan had in mind. It did, however, suit the pecuniary needs of the other partners. They did not like her style, but tolerated her on account of the financial rewards to the practice. This outlook was even further diminished when James broke his leg overseas and required multiple operations, leaving him away from the centre for many months. Also, Kennan had his rooms moved to a wing of the practice, along with a supportive psychology colleague. They were being deliberately marginalised to the main thrust of the centre.

Even these changes Kennan managed. But because James was away from work for this significant period, his influence was negligible. He decided to ride the storm. Yet the staff atmosphere also started to deteriorate and eventually one receptionist, well known to and supportive of Kennan, but alienated from others by the manageress, suicided. The wheels started to come off. Kennan started to develop a migraine syndrome that affected his nervous system functioning and … his alcohol intake started to rise.

As these events continued inexorably, it seemed, Kennan had discussions with his pharmacy friend, Thomas, who now ran HealthQuest. Whilst at Mandurah, Kennan had maintained the friendship and support of HealthQuest by doing an occasional session there. After all, it was only 60 kilometres to the city. With the events unfolding, Thomas, who was now also unhappy with the clinic's direction, had discussions with Kennan about setting up a new clinic according to Kennan's original ideas.

Kennan had resisted these overtures, but as things started to unravel at the centre in Mandurah, he turned his attention back to Thomas. But he realised this was futile as the business plans couldn't bear fruit, and he pulled the plug on both the speculation and his occasional presence at HealthQuest. Mandurah may have been in a relatively early and immature state from his perspective, but he felt he was better off putting all his attention to the one project. With this, I would finally agree, although I don't know whether I would have persisted with the Mandurah clinic the way it was going!

In some ways, Kennan seems to have relatively large blind spots in his psychological makeup; I am sure these could be psychologically labelled, but I don't feel that is simply the case. This is the deeper more-fated directive that seems to grip him and make him try to push through regardless. He might not have wanted to be a martyr, but he was headed in that direction; sometimes his 'gods' seem to me to be quite dark at the personal level.

To date, alcohol had not directly influenced Kennan's work, or so he thought. He did not drink before or during working hours, and had kept this as a personal rule. To avoid this potential possibility, he started to use the occasional sedative, first at night, but then sometimes a small portion of a pill during the day to cope with the nervous system symptoms; but also, to my mind, to cope with the stresses and isolation.

In the last week Kennan was to work at the centre, he missed one day because of illness, did half days for a couple, and then came in one afternoon having had a couple of drinks at lunchtime following a sedative in the early hours of the morning. The manageress smelled the alcohol on his breath when they spoke and reported this to one of the partners. On Peter's request, he went home.

"Is this the only time you have had a drink and gone to work?" I asked.

"No," he replied. I wanted to believe otherwise when I had asked the question, but I was not surprised by the answer.

"I think you have adequately explained how you got to this

point; but with the wisdom of hindsight, where does alcohol fit in?"

Kennan took a deep breath. "Things got out of control in the months prior, when I started to develop the nervous system problems. It was kind of downhill from there."

"Surely you shared this with someone?" I countered.

"Of course, I did, with James. He was now back at work but not fully functional. I discussed the symptoms in detail and we had a plan of action, until the above event superseded."

"So, he knew about the alcohol?"

"Yes. I had come to work affected a few months before, but didn't see any patients. If I was trying to hide a habit, I would have done a helluva better job, as I know others did and still do. James knew I was overdoing it, but it was a rare occasion I'd have a drink in the day to settle my nerves, maybe three or four times in total, and usually in the early evening to get through a late surgery. On this occasion, I was really and unusually unwell; also, I was behind with my patient load because of the missed time earlier in the week, and I made a choice and used champagne as a kind of pick-me-up. A very poor choice, as it turns out, or an ideal one, considering how I feel now."

Kennan needed to explain this last comment to me. In summary, he indicated that there was obviously a powerful inner unseen urge to leave medical practice, and this sequence of events proved ideal, although this was only a very vague understanding at the time. He obviously had a different take on the forces driving him than my earlier deduction.

I asked him if it was actually a choice then?

"A choice to drink? Yes. To leave? No ... well it didn't appear to be so until some days later."

"What happened?"

"Well, I immediately took leave and pulled myself together. I decided to have a break and get to the bottom of the symptoms before I returned, and I also decided to not have further alcohol – at all – if I continued in practice."

"But that's not how things turned out, is it?"

"No," he replied. "At the next partners' meeting, it was decided to refer the situation to the medical practitioner's governing body, the Medical Board, through a supervening governing agency called the Australian Health Practitioners Regulation Authority, or AHPRA. This was as a result of one of the partners phoning a Medical Board colleague who informed her that working under the influence of alcohol required mandatory notification to AHPRA. There was nothing James could now do to shield me so, with my knowledge, he notified AHPRA. Then events unfolded very, or too rapidly; meaning that I suspect there were agendas operating behind the scenes that I can only guess at and may never know, although some seem to be revealing themselves over time. Interestingly, they match my impressions with the exception of one – sexual jealousy." I made a mental note of this. It seemed Kennan is on the edge of a particularly significant blind spot.

"What transpired from this was that AHPRA decided that, if I were to continue practice then, they would conduct an investigation, and also a personal health review not of my choosing, whilst I worked in a restricted capacity. This judgement was unilateral. I was not seen, consulted or talked to then, or subsequently, so my current health circumstances were never elucidated. Of course, they would have been over time, but in the meantime, I was guilty of being an alcoholic until proven innocent. I have since found that this is common draconian institutionalism, and that there are many doctors who continue to practice under similar, or even worse restricted circumstances, until such time as they clear themselves or they recover from their health concerns. AHPRA have become a law unto themselves; in fact, even the Federal Government has little say over their actions."

"So, why aren't you still practising? Why didn't you take that option?"

"As I was being told this by my medical defence lawyer, who seemed quite powerless in this circumstance now with AHPRA's input, I looked out of the window from the third floor down a really attractive tree-lined mews that wound its way behind some houses across the road. I suddenly saw that I had been instrumental in what had happened, in a way that gave me an option to leave practice totally and finally, and that this was what was being asked of me."

"By your 'gods' I presume?" At this stage, I was not being sarcastic.

"Yes, in a way, but it was more an intuition then. It was like someone showing me another path, another option. I had summoned this with my actions, the alcohol, and the illness I was experiencing. I also 'saw' that if I didn't leave then I would continue in practice and be another statistic. I would be dead. And AHPRA didn't give a shit. They were hiding behind their "protecting the public interest" line. But what about me? The closest anyone got to contacting me was the Medical Board doctor who had been rung originally. After he heard that I had resigned, he rang James to find out if I was okay. I think he was frightened I may have killed myself!"

"So that was the point you resigned?"

"Yes. I turned around and told this to my lawyer and a counselling doctor who was also present at the meeting I had initiated independently about my situation, when the AHPRA edict was phoned through, coincidentally – or so it seemed – at the same time. The doctor didn't understand why I would voluntarily give up medical practice, but the lawyer got it – she knew why. They had their hands tied too, I guess.

"I then went home to consider for a few days, and to discuss with my wife and others, before formally resigning. I looked at my actions, what I had done, and where it was leading me. I saw that I had chosen to escape and was responsible for my actions, even if indirectly or subconsciously.

"I could see how the partners were gutless in the face of the dominance of the manageress; they were seduced by her appeal to their hip pockets. I could also see how they were threatened by what I was doing, and there was more than a streak of jealousy in many. But mainly I saw that they were moral cowards, in spite of all the so-called 'political correctness'.

"Some years later, I was to put another piece of the jigsaw puzzle in when I was told that there were dynamics of sex and power, including using me in some sort of payback manner, which had been involved in the partners' decision-making. This was an accidental finding with a large slice of innuendo embedded in it, so I won't unpack this part of the story any further." And that's as far as Kennan would go in committing the undercurrents to this record.

"My card was most certainly already 'marked' with the institutions, and the price of continued practice would continue to be draconian. I could see that in spite of being a 'family practice' that also supposedly had the concern of their staff at the forefront, as often espoused by one of the senior partners, they were ultimately concerned for their own welfare. The receptionist's suicide had alerted me to this. But, above all these issues, I saw that I was being pointed in another direction."

We followed this with a long discussion about the role of the authorities in the healthcare field, which was a matter of mutual concern. We both agreed that their influence in medicine was heavily politicised and economically driven; that there were too many governing bodies with excessive power, with the net effect healthcare in general and particularly medicine was greatly diminished as a consequence. And, irrespective of all the rhetoric about public safety and interest, it was now a largely fascist structure, in Kennan's opinion. I was starting to agree with the starkness and implications of this viewpoint.

"I was once told by a lawyer, who also held medical degrees, that challenging the Medical Board and AHPRA was like dealing with a rabid dog!" Kennan smiled as he recounted this story.

"And you feel that was your experience?" I countered.

"Well, yes; effectively a Star Chamber, or a kangaroo court, in my view," he replied. "But I really had to and have been building my future around the significance of the event, and where it is directing me."

"You're being a bit cryptic and, I sense, metaphoric?"

"Well, let's put this episode, in context, to bed, so to speak, and get on with issues of more significance and importance. This may be my perspective, but it is more important to see health and medicine in a much broader context than the one defined and controlled by the institutions and their political masters.

"Medicine is an art and a craft. A doctor's license should follow a proper apprenticeship and be the passport to practice medicine as and in whatever way he or she sees fit. This should be based primarily on the contract between doctor and patient, not evidence and protocols. And, just to throw some petrol on the fire, some of my best 'medicine' has been when I've had a couple of drinks; out of formal practice, of course.

"We are in an era where institutionalisation reigns. We have lost the perspective where the rules and laws result from contracts, or negotiations between people that lead to the rules that govern them and their behaviour. Instead, the institutions have become detached from those they purport to serve, yet hypocritically claim they represent the interests of the so-called public. It is, in my naïve view, somewhat fascist. It hides behind the illusion – delusion – of democracy and we, the general public, have fallen for it."

I interjected: "So why haven't you tried to change this system from the inside?"

"Because in my own way I have tried, but I don't believe it can be done." He paused for a lengthy time. "And, I do not believe it is my path. Let me tell you a story: Just before my 21st birthday I was walking down a street in Oxford heading back to college. It was late at night, but still relatively busy. I turned into a road and in front of me were three young men. They were obviously not students and were loud, and maybe the worse for wear. They took up the footpath in such a way that I would have to step around them, maybe onto the road, to get past. I chose not to and heavily brushed shoulders with the outside man of the group.

"I walked on, but heard them turn around and follow me. The man I brushed pulled me around and punched me in the head. I fell to the ground. As I raised my head to get up, I saw a boot coming toward it. Then pain and confusion followed as the other men pulled him away and ran off. Blood was pouring from my nose and I got to my feet to find myself surrounded by several people, mainly students, a few of whom I knew.

"I leaned back against a wall and felt my nose, it seemed loose and misshapen, but I was not too concerned and straightened it a bit. I was taken to the local hospital where a very sympathetic doctor showed me my nose in a mirror. I was shocked to see it across and flattened against one side of my face. I wondered what it must have been like before my own earlier attempt to straighten it."

""You have two choices," the doctor said, "I can patch you up and book you in for a surgical correction in a few days. Or, I can try and straighten it now."

"I took the latter option. He painted the inside of my nose with cocaine and then proceeded to wrench it across. Twice. He took me back to the mirror and my nose was straight. We shook hands and I departed to go and lick my wounds. My assailants were never found and I ultimately received some compensation for a criminal injury, which I used to buy a new stereo system. It was called the 'golden nose award' by my friends! The doctor did a good job, nobody can tell the bridge of my nose has been shattered, unless they feel the lumps under the skin."

I could have responded with questions, but now being used to Kennan's style, I knew this story would unravel.

"My situation was then, and still being, mine to deal with. Sure, the institutions are callous and uncaring, but they are what they are. I confronted them and made an error of judgement in the process. I received my just reward knowing my card was marked, probably as a trouble-maker. But I also wanted it over with quickly; I didn't want a protracted process around responsibility and justice, when both are palpably lacking, hypocritical, and essentially false. As such, the process lasted a week instead of years. I wanted to get on, now that it was apparent to me that I had deliberately wagged the tail of the rabid dog.

"That the situation was very messy, and people like James were compromised, there is no doubt. And that there was a fair amount of threat and fear also being dealt with by the partners at the centre, my own medical defence people and maybe others, I have equally no doubt. But these people were playing by the rules of a game they themselves had inherited, and there was no room to change the contract, to negotiate any variation. This was not just in regard to my own situation; it was also with my greater concern for medicine and its direction.

"I have progressively been of the opinion that the changes to medicine, the transition and hopefully transformation, will come from the emerging community consciousness. It will be the will of the recipients of healthcare delivery who will instigate the changes."

I was obvious to me, the alcohol notwithstanding, that Kennan's health had been a prior source of concern and instrumental in the events that unfolded. Kennan told me that, with James's assistance, he rapidly unpacked his symptoms. They were a direct result of the stress pattern. James, an expert in addiction, had always maintained that Kennan was not an alcoholic, but had a significant post-traumatic stress disorder, or PTSD that he was negotiating in an unhealthy way.

Kennan's adrenal glands were working overtime, according to testing, and were to come back down to normal within weeks of stopping medical practice; a statement in and of itself. His blood sugar levels were erratic during this period, again as a result of stress, but also explained his predilection to drink white wine or champagnes and not his favoured red, when stressed. And, there was no further surprise that the neurological symptoms abated during the same period, and have not returned years later.

What is it that our doctors get so ill? Why aren't they cared for? I am sure the answers to this are embedded in this account, as well as my own experience of them. Not only are they stressed and pressured, they are also isolated and unsupported. And the various institutions that claim to take account for this and care evidently do not. In Kennan's case, once he resigned, nobody in the profession, except James and couple of his doctor friends from elsewhere, showed any interest. It is an irony that the supposed institutional care of the public does not afford their professionals the same consideration. The problem of Kennan was solved, end of story.

What most practitioners, and some other healthcare professionals he knew, were more interested in was the choice he had made; it was as if they didn't feel they had an option, and therefore reflected the opinion of the doctor present at Kennan's lawyer meeting. Without exception, they considered his decision brave, and most expressed envy. This surprised him. When challenged about their own choice to stay under this duress, he received the predictable responses of marriage, mortgage, school fees, and the like. Yet Kennan was to unravel some interesting facts. He found that a significant number, easily the majority he knew, had or were having difficulties with the authorities. Most kept this to themselves; it wasn't a good advertisement, after all! Yet even he was surprised at the percentage.

What was interesting about the complaints that practitioners he knew were subject to was that none came from a patient. This was Kennan's experience; as stated already, he had never been the subject of a patient complaint. So where had they come from? Well, they had either come from colleagues, or referrals to the various Boards and hence the supervening AHPRA from other institutional authorities, such as the courts. In a couple of cases he examined, he suspected legal pursuit. In other words, they were vexatious. The conclusions from this brief survey seemed obvious to Kennan and he decided it was not in his emotional interest, with a view to the grieving he was about to go through, to delve any further.

Similarly, the notifications for issues like alcohol and drugs are distorted. Doctors work in a variety of circumstances – for example, if Kennan had been a partner of the centre's practice, then maybe the manageress' report would have been dealt with internally? If she or another who noticed were an employee of the practitioner, would they raise a complaint? As complaints could be anonymous, isn't the reporting system itself open to abuse?

Kennan's appreciation of the use of alcohol amongst practitioners increased, now he was not simply watching himself and his own potential exposure. Similarly, he was to discover a prevalence amongst them for the use of drugs of prescription.

His own sparse use, although only with the culminating event of his career, declined and ceased with his symptom relief. Yet he discovered the use of agents such as anti-anxiety and anti-depressants to be significant and concerning amongst the profession at large. He also hinted at significant illicit drug usage, but declined to go further.

My feeling is that, in line with his account of the Oxford assault, Kennan had taken responsibility for what happened to him, as well as the consequences. Although traumatised by the event, he was not surprised about what he was almost inadvertently uncovering.

Before we finished with this episode, I asked Kennan how he would have handled the situation, should it have been presented to him, knowing that he had been in a medical partnership in the past.

"In the past, the Medical Board would triage problems; that is, assign them a certain priority, and often dismiss or sideline the trivial, I guess. With the creation of a supervening institution like AHPRA, this has changed and all complaints are investigated, or so we are told. The problem with this is that this is open to vexatious and anonymous complaints. As I have indicated, personally I have yet to hear of a case where the source is a patient; it is more likely to be a colleague or an associated agency. Also, AHPRA's powers are considerable and relatively unfettered; its judgements are unilateral, and not appealable. It may also be that institutions like this attract those who have a vested psychological interest in pursuing and controlling doctors.

"So, any alternative requires a risk on behalf of others, in my own case the centre partners. The call to the Board member in the first place, I would not have agreed with. In the company of the partners, I would have discussed the situation with Kennan – myself – and outlined a plan of action. This would have included the management of his apparent illness to a satisfactory conclusion, which would mean practice adjustment and even jointly planning his future.

"Could James have done this?" I asked.

"Feasibly, but unlikely as he was away from the centre at the time in question and not involved in the incident. The phone call sealed the situation as it created an obligation, which I suspect the partner making the call already knew. Maybe we just have a slight difference in our attitude toward authority and the situation polarised this."

"You don't disrespect James as a result?"

"No. We are all adults and take responsibility for ourselves and have to deal with the consequences of our actions. James did what he thought was best at the time, I guess. If he were on his own in the decision-making, he may well have kept the situation in-house and managed it accordingly. It is the manageress, some of the partners, and their personal interests that I have contempt for and would take issue with."

I'm not sure whether the bulk of this chapter will have a wide appeal, except to health professionals. However, I do believe the general public should understand the unseen patterns that exist behind the health and medical practice that is delivered to them. In my experience, most do not know much about the governing agencies that are meant to serve them.

I wondered whether Kennan would at some stage return to practice. This did not cross Kennan's mind; he was finished with medical practice. He obviously retains his medical degrees and will always be a doctor of medicine. He had a therapeutic clientele that would now simply not come under the domain of mental health as in medical practice. This effectively meant that clients would not get rebates, and he would also no longer have to imply that the therapy was directed toward treatment for a defined mental health illness. Rather, it was and is directed toward self-discovery and personal growth, and can now be conducted more adventurously. He does not now see his work as primarily therapeutic, or therapeutically directed, as commonly understood.

There were also his books. Indeed, it had been the writing of one a few months before he resigned that might have had an impact on the subsequent drama and where he now found himself. This was an account of the spirituality of the Anglo-Saxon or Old English period and an analysis of the runes – symbols that were and still are used for magic, healing and divination. The manuscript had received acceptance abroad and was subsequently published in Britain, along with one of his earlier works.

Writing this particular book had a significant impact: it turned Kennan's attention to that period's view of medicine and the management of health in a way that he believed had modern application, particularly for mental health. He also experienced, for the first time in his life, a view of death that did not carry the doubts and fears he had hitherto held. It was like an epiphany; this was an area he wanted to immerse himself in.

Maybe his blind spots congeal around a core apparent death wish that reflects his attraction to medicine? But not only his, but all professionals in the field. If so, then that – as Kennan suspects – is the bedrock flaw in the foundation of modern western medicine, something he has more than hinted at variously in this account.

Is this pattern the one that stands behind the trauma and sabotage he has undergone? Is it an act of self-sacrifice to a higher good? Is this what needs to happen to the profession at large so that it can renew itself?

But, at this point in his account, it was the grief of losing a career that spanned nearly four decades and how to negotiate the future that preoccupied him. There was still bread to put on the table and the deeper question of what was being asked of him in the spiritual sense.

Fourteen

It is nearly eight years since Kennan left medicine and we are now up to date with the chronology, although I suspect unravelling this last period may offer some surprises. At a conscious and practical level, I doubt whether Kennan ever saw that he would be outside of the medical fraternity. It is not what medical doctors who become practitioners usually do; in fact, I know of no other medical practitioner who has taken this step, unless it is to pursue an alternative career.

However, once registered, they usually remain so, even if not in practice, which Kennan could have done. The other unusual factor is that he could still work in his chosen field, except in an unregistered capacity. To be honest to this change, the rebranding process would be away from medical practitioner, specifically being a medical psychotherapist in Kennan's case. Instead, he was free to ally his therapeutic work more with his spiritual orientation now as a mentor and teacher.

What did he lose in this move? He could no longer prescribe or order investigations, but that was insignificant in practice, as colleagues could and would undertake this along with the attendant responsibilities. He also lost a lot of stress. What he gained was freedom of expression, and as his vocation as a wordsmith was increasingly coming to the fore, to be unfettered in what he could say about health was a distinct advantage.

Yet, to my mind at least, there was and is something deeper and more powerful operating within Kennan. He is very much his own man, a marginal person, and seemed to me to be struggling to access something within the broader field of medicine that he felt the modern era lacks. While he had tried to keep this impetus contained in parallel interests, it seems that, initiated by and beyond the events culminating some eight years ago, he can no longer contain himself. In fact, the desire for this emergence was and is more powerful than his attempts to keep it in control. This is not an uncommon dynamic in life, it seems; a kind of breakthrough or now with an arrow that only goes in one direction.

Maybe I was also gaining an appreciation of how these forces work, to be able to see them operating this way within Kennan, as well as myself, of course! Both of us are well aware that this level and way of understanding is foreign, even alien to our day-to-day and materialistic reality. But it helps explain a lot to me, not only in his case, but in other theatres of the world. These observations and conclusions we shared between ourselves because Kennan had gained an unequivocal perspective of himself and how he must operate in society at large.

I think this was touched on a little earlier with the concept of the daimon. As I understand it, further to the earlier exposition, this is an inner inspiring force that operates within an individual and can be seen as embodying the relationship between the supernatural – in whatever way we individually view it – and man. It could be reflected in such terms as destiny, fate, or even soul. It is easy to see how this concept has become 'demonised' within Christianity, as the arrogance of considering such an individual relationship with the divine is considered hubris by the conventional Church.

There are three points that might help explain this a little further. The first is the idea that we are living in a kind of cultural flatland – being a metaphor for the lack of depth we experience in the present era. We live in a world that lacks its full dimensionality. Most obvious, this is the case with religion, which no longer holds its thrall. Our inherent spirituality – our depth – is wandering rudderless and poorly recognised, attaching itself to false gods, like science, which then becomes a religious 'scientism' that taints such as the medical profession.

The second is that Kennan progressively came to understand that he was living a shamanic existence. One of the central tenets of shamanism is that healing can be a calling or vocation, and that not following the calling can lead one into darkness, disease, or even death. Alternatively, it could be seen that illness and disease could be the initiator for the shamanic way of life, a healing vocation. It doesn't take much consideration from this point to ask oneself whether all illness and disease has their basis in the shamanic worldview.

The third is the inherent difference and potential conflict between the individual who realises and enacts the above, and the demands of duty and obligation, from whatever sources. Adherence to the first essentially makes one who follows such a path an 'outsider' and prey to the criticism, blame and judgement from the majority who follow the conventional paths laid down by the establishment of the time. The outcome for such an individual is hardly an easy existence. The paradox is that this same individual may be setting the tone for future norms. The difference here between sacrifice and martyrdom in this domain can be subtle.

It could be tedious to go through the account of this period up to the present in any further detail. In an emotional context, life's personal journey is for the individual, only more broadly relevant if what is learned or discovered has wider application and significance, and then conveyed best by narrative. Kennan was of the same opinion when we met to discuss this period, so he left me to ask questions or lead the conversation into areas that I would consider of interest to the reader.

Kennan maintained that it took a few years to feel clear of

medicine, the institution. Did this mean that prior to this time he had a secret longing to return? He maintained this was not the case, except as a kind of undercurrent when finances became difficult, which they were for most of this period. Suddenly and without preparation to have a significant source of income no longer coming in was a shock to the family, particularly as the decision was of his own choosing. His marriage weathered this, and his wife was a support, but it came close to the edge on several occasions and ultimately, as we shall see, it was to dissolve.

The last threatening event was when Kennan decided to mortgage his home retreat property of Ganieda in the south and use the funds to invest in a business unrelated to the health industry. Without a cash flow of note, it was a very difficult time, so when the opportunity arose he trusted his feeling, such that the dividends from the business would provide some flexibility. However, I suspect that he agreed there was too much fear in the decision and that his deeper intuition was saying otherwise. Even though he maintained a psychotherapy practice during this period he put little effort into it, which surprised him. He felt that even this avenue was closing or at least changing, irrespective of the adjustments in perspective he had taken with it.

I found this a little difficult to understand, as Kennan now had any psychotherapy directed exclusively toward self-discovery and personal growth, rather than taking a mental health and hence illness orientation. This was a natural thread to continue beyond medicine, as it harkened back to his days as a Jungian analyst. Most people who maintained contact with him during this transition understood this, because in many ways it was not significantly different to the actual way he had practised any therapy within the medical context.

Psychotherapy was a minor though valuable source of

income, however, so Kennan maintained it; although more as a barometer of where he was actually heading ... which was where? What was emerging was a more mentoring and teaching theme to his work. Any advice or counselling he gave was of a more educational nature. He was also approached to do health-oriented seminars by various people and he took the opportunity to extend these into workshops on occasion, where therapy was a natural consequence, but not the primary intent or focus.

Earlier, Kennan had eschewed any direction toward teaching and training. In his own career development, he experienced formal teachers to be generally failed practitioners, with the exception of his clinical training in London, where successful practitioners were the teachers. Yet there seemed to be a tendency for people in the health and personal development fields to want to develop a teaching and training focus at an early opportunity, often prematurely, it seemed to him. He reasoned that most of this was financial, and he understood this, but his interest and direction in medicine had always been as a practitioner.

It was this reality that hurt most: Kennan still felt himself to be a very good diagnostician; he had learned his art well. So, to have that 'right' of formal medical practice removed, even though voluntarily, was difficult. This was particularly so when he witnessed the progressive scientific dominance of medicine, with its attendant objectification and, in his mind, dehumanisation. It was also common in his social circle to encounter people who had fallen through the diagnostic cracks of modern western medicine and were either not cared for or experiencing inappropriate management as a result.

Progressively, Kennan started to appreciate that a teaching framework offered many advantages because he did now see himself more as an educator or, more correctly, a teacher. Anything that could be seen as diagnostic, therapeutic, or practice readily flowed from this. And now, because the framework he was using was health, specifically holistic health, he felt he had moved beyond any difficulties around conflict with the medical profession.

As he explained it: "Modern medicine is based on disease and pathology. It is scientific and mechanical, deals with physical dysfunction, and even mistakenly sees the mind and mental health as a mere extension of a bodily organ, the brain. Holism, as we've referred to many times in this account, is more physiologically than pathologically based. It sees problems and illness as a variation of normal and capable of rectification, even self-rectification, prior to taking over control with the treatment that ensues from a modern medical perspective.

"Authentic holistic health sees things differently to modern medicine. There is the body and the inner more subtle world of emotions, mind and intellect. There is the outer social world, with its environmental, occupational and familial extensions. Then there is the spiritual perspective that embraces and supervenes all of this. Modern medicine occupies a place in this overall scheme of things, but as you can see by the way I have described it, it is a rather limited one.

"As you know, it is my belief that medicine must transition to and even reinvent itself in this broader – holistic – perspective; this is a paradigm shift that is already in process, even if this is early days. But before we get to how this might look, what I recognised I needed to do a while ago was put myself firmly in that holistic picture and operate from there. And that this was as a teacher, including education and training, but fundamentally as a teacher, healer and mentor in the traditional sense."

This is a summary I will ask him to return to in a different context before we finish. Like other topics in this account that repeat themselves, it is because they can be viewed not only in different contexts for a fuller understanding, but they also mean different things to Kennan at the various stages of his own development. These concepts should be seen as fluid and evolving, not fixed and static.

Kennan's account of the last few years post-medicine showed the trend he describes slowly emerging. There were some cul-de-sacs and rabbit holes, predictably, but the twin themes of holism and teaching became progressively stronger. However, the process hadn't been completely integrated and become consolidated, and there were two themes that led to this happening.

The first was a consequence of the marital stress when he decided to invest in the business that was to supply the family cash flow, but nonetheless seemed a risky move. Following a short overseas trip to Bali with the other shareholders in this business, Kennan and his wife were to return with what seemed like colds. Kennan had developed the viral pneumonia that occurred early in our meetings and which I shared in an earlier chapter, but would like to elaborate on further. He knew antibiotics would be of little help and probably be harmful, so he simply went into a hibernation of sorts. It was a painful time. What affected him most was his complete loss of any volition. It seemed to him that his willpower and intent to do anything at all had simply evaporated; everything was just too hard.

The illness itself did not seem unusual. I think he was right in his self-diagnosis and respect his choice not to undertake any pharmaceutical management, apart from occasional analgesics. I don't think he was being reckless; it was just unusual management from a contemporary perspective, although in keeping with his nature and a consequence of the deep feeling he had that this illness marked some sort of transition.

However, the weakness and lack of volition were intense, and were also clues of a kind to Kennan. He felt that his body was going through some sort of readjustment and that the lack of will, not unusual in severe illness, was to allow this deeper healing to proceed. He tells me that, unlike other illness he has had, there was a deep trust in this process and that, whilst concerned, he never felt frightened.

There was another significant factor in this illness. Kennan's alcohol intake, whilst relatively stable and considerably reduced following his exit from medicine, started to escalate over this stressful time of the business acquisition, in a pattern that concerned both he and his wife. So, two months prior to this illness, he had ceased drinking completely, something that continued for a period of six months and embraced the pneumonia. He felt there was a detoxification going on in the illness, or that it was even its purpose. This was something that could not easily be proven, but it remains his conviction.

Alcohol has now returned to Kennan's life, but the potential binges that marked the last few years are now absent. He tells me that he feels this is permanent, unless, of course, he wished to leave the planet. I looked up, concerned, but he was already smiling back at me. When he does or says things like this, I don't know whether to laugh or hit him!

It was after this illness that Kennan started to feel that any formal psychotherapy would eventually fade out of his professional picture. Over the previous two years he had assembled, along with colleagues on occasion, a package of educational material around holistic health and in a variety of formats. He had conducted pilot groups of a training nature and started to structure all this work into a more formal educational format.

Yet, in spite of his best endeavours, the material could be seen as simply some sort of expansion of, or complement to the status quo of modern medicine. This concerned Kennan, but he was not sure where to take it. He felt that, in some way, what he was offering was still some sort of 'apologetic' position to scientific medicine, and that the majority of the public would perceive it that way.

Kennan knew the solution, but had, to this point, erred on the side of caution. He needed to focus on the second theme of the integration process. And, if truth be told, he had known about this all along. It started to emerge with the work he was doing in the south at Ganieda, which he still saw as his future home again and where the development caused him to regularly visit from Perth to attend to this, either in an administrative, or an active and physical manner.

Whilst back there, Kennan reconnected with the prior development conducted in the many years when he had lived there, and it all had a deep impression on him. The spirituality of the land and what he had constructed to date was drawing him back in, and this time without family expectation. It was a challenging focus. He picked up on the themes in a book he wrote the year he left medical practice, about the runes and Anglo-Saxon spirituality. The core theme that emerged from his research into the creation of the book was around Anglo-Saxon or Old English medicine, and specifically that prior to the Norman conquest of 1066.

I was more than a little curious. It seemed to me that the actual writing had been very evocative, that much was apparent. But had it also been 'invocative', and called forth his ancestral past? Had a Pandora's box of issues been opened or unearthed in such a way that he couldn't or wouldn't put the lid back on? Although these comments could be seen as metaphoric, I was a little unsettled; could they also be literally true? Certainly, Kennan suspected – now – that this was a likely scenario. And why was this?

We shared and discussed the content of the book, which was

a reconstruction of Heathen Britain prior to and beneath the Christian religious conversion. Christianisation had occurred in progressive waves after the Romans left in the 5th century, to become the dominant religious and political force that we know today. But as a social force Christianity had not been as successful and, at some level, it had and has never fully succeeded – this was all in Kennan's opinion, and as reflected in his deeper childhood experience.

Psychically it was a big task and emotional challenge for Kennan to strip away his own personal Christianisation. In many ways, this had occurred during his adventures into Jungian analysis, alternative healing, and the new age generally. But this time it was different; it seemed like his Heathen ancestry had been summoned, or was summoning him and was more powerful than his ability to resist. He found in the medicine of that time a significantly different pattern of belief, application, and practice. It was also in contrast to the Mediterranean medicine that has become the cultural foundation of modern western medicine.

"What made or makes it so different?" I asked.

Kennan found it difficult to explain in detail: "It's a task I have just started on again," he explained, indicating an anticipated and committed future. "It is deeply rooted in the environment and the Heathen belief system. It connects with the gods and other beings the Anglo-Saxons and their predecessors, the Celts, accepted as part of their life. It is deeply imbued with magical practice and with a medicine of spells and rituals, not unlike the North American Indian and their medicine men."

I got the picture, vaguely. I nuanced his account slightly: "So, is it shamanic?"

"You're getting good," Kennan responded, smirking. "We'll make a medicine man out of you yet!" I think he was actually serious though ...

There were other themes. "When I began to look at the runes in a bit more detail, I started to see there was a pattern in the Anglo-Saxon runes that differed from the other Germanic and Scandinavian rune systems. There was an extension of sorts that connected back to the pre-migration era; that is, the Celtic world of Britain that existed prior to and within the Roman occupation period. And there was an extension the other way, beyond and different from the other rune systems, which was subtly influenced by Christianity, or that Christianity appropriated from a prior Heathen influence.

"However, this wasn't the Christianity that we now know, it was a mystical thread that emerged centuries later in the second millennium in the Arthurian and Holy Grail legends. It is also deeply connected to alchemy, or a proto-alchemy that stretches back to the dawn of historical time with megalithic stones and blacksmiths. So, all this is mixed up – in my mind anyway – with the medicine of that period, and paints a remarkably different picture to the one that resides in the history books."

All I could really do was listen. I was in no position to comment beyond a point, either to discuss, or criticise. It was all news to me, but it all did seem to hang together; it certainly did in Kennan's mind. But I could see the integrative pattern in his consciousness and its imaginative extension.

Kennan went on to tell me that this whole area is now his life's work, and he calls it shamanic or soul medicine. He is supported by some other people in this, from therapeutic, academic and teaching fields. He also explained to me that this has added a possible place for his retreat home, Ganieda, into the future, as well as also an open-ended extension to his work in holistic health delivery. In his account of this he sees that the teaching and training he intends to offer in holistic health connects organically to this larger field of inquiry and is embedded in it, rather than being simply some sort of counterbalance to the deficiencies of modern medicine.

So, where to from here for this man? Maybe this is best understood by laying out his current professional profile, before discussing the shortfalls of modern western medicine in some detail, and then moving to some speculation about where modern medicine goes from this point on. Kennan considers this last step to be at least a transition and maybe – hopefully – a transformation. But he also sees it deeply embedded in a holistic perspective that includes the inner and outer worlds, mind and body, which is where his current working profile resides.

Kennan no longer sees himself as a practitioner in the health field. From a medical perspective, this was renounced several years ago, but its significance is wider. Practice infers treatment, and medicine is about diagnosis and treatment. As modern treatment is mechanically and physically-based, Kennan had no difficulty parting company here. With diagnosis this is different, as he does not see that as institutional medicine's right; it is more of an art, in his opinion.

Initially, Kennan simply picked up the threads of his mental health work and restructured it privately, in the manner already discussed. He found and finds the term 'analyst' anachronistic and incorrect, and 'psychotherapist' to be a misnomer, although to the modern mentality it still best describes how he works. But he also sees modern psychology, as a discipline, to have appropriated and misrepresented the Greek word psyche, or soul. He didn't and still doesn't care much for psychology either in its various academic, research and clinical forms.

What emerged over this period was actually no professional title at all. Kennan simply provided a health consultancy that included counselling and therapy, as well as teaching and mentorship. As we have already discussed, the title of teacher became maybe the most appropriate title for him to use, should he be inclined; but he wasn't particularly, as another awaited him. I must add that he tends to take me to task with my emphasis around teaching and education, as he does not see it that way and merely an attempt on my behalf to buttonhole him into a category that I feel comfortable with. There may be more than a grain of truth in his perception here ...

From a medical perspective, Kennan was fortunate to have at least two colleagues to refer to, who both understood and supported him. In this way, he felt he was an addition to the medical system in his new role, but was sure the institution may not consider it that way! It afforded him the privilege of stating that he did not provide registered medical or health practitioner services, and so to lead his clientele away from establishment viewpoints. In the area of mental health, in particular, he saw this as most valuable.

Kennan was to see that even this framework was and is a transition. As the philosophical, humanistic (I had written 'educational' here, but he crossed it out and entered 'humanistic' instead!) and spiritual dimensions of his work become the preferred background, he feels that any future consultancy work would increasingly come from this developing culture. This lacked many of the concerns that offering a different framework and perspective presented to potential clientele. In effect, either they appreciated it and the services offered, or they did not. Selection became increasingly self-directed and simplified.

As did the setting: there was no need for reception or undue administration, in fact they could be a hindrance to healing work. His work was now not the subject of the prying eyes of the establishment or even the direct purview of such as the legal profession. Kennan could work from his lounge room, phone, or online video. He could sit with a client on a park bench, at a café, or go on a walk with them. The options became more creative and genuinely therapeutic or, as he preferred to call it, healing.

Any counselling education and training is a different matter. Here the relationship with the teacher, mentor and/or supervisor is essential. So, Kennan has developed a highly personal and idiosyncratic method of teaching people to be holistic counsellors or become a medicine man/woman. As he also attracts potential students with extensive life experience and personal preferences, he has found a way to integrate this, as well as ways to do this on an individual basis.

Yet neither of these streams of education and training would have held his attention without the spiritual dimension. As we have discussed and returned to on several occasions, it is a ready-made trap for anyone offering a difference to mainstream medicine and psychology to undertake either a complementary approach, or become an alternative to it. Either way is disempowering; it still acknowledges mainstream as the standard to be measured against, and Kennan is at pains to point out that this may no longer be the case. Yet he also needed to position himself in a way that clearly demonstrates his belief; he needed to walk his talk.

Maybe his home retreat had been premature, an intuition of what could be. In Kennan's words though, he hoped it did not end up "like Camelot!" referring to the mythic demise of that focus of spirituality within the world. I wondered why, when it seemed to be headed in that direction, that Kennan chose to leave his southern home on two occasions. He explained to me the circumstances, which we have already covered, but now as some sort of journey to arrive at where he now stood.

Standing was probably the wrong term; the man was and is fluid. In between his journeys toward and away from home and the land of the deep south, Kennan had much to learn and digest. He feels he was now ready and that home, or an alternative, is waiting. As an extension of his work, he has always believed spiritual retreat to be a core intense focus for healing and personal transformation. He now counts himself as part of the process.

The home retreat of Ganieda lay expectant, awaiting input and progress. In his ideas and imagination, Kennan centres himself there, as well visiting for increasing periods of personal retreat, reflection, and direction. He involves himself in a physical and practical way with its maintenance. In the past, he built a sweat lodge underground, a development of the North American Indian model, but adapted to his Anglo-Saxon and Celtic heritage (which he now refers to as 'Anglo-Celtic'). There was also a ceremonial stone circle of some ten metres diameter to work with, in a ritual spiritual sway, as well as to provide healing ceremonies.

In his inner world, things have settled considerably. Kennan feels in a different place to even before the pneumonia. As with all significant illness he has experienced this had a changing and sustained effect on him; he feels it still. There is no going back, so what does going forward look like? He seemed unable or reluctant to answer that question. Rather, he talked of where he sees himself now.

Kennan is developing a body of work he calls Soul Medicine. This flows on from a diploma course he developed with a colleague some twenty years ago, called Traditional Medicine Ways. The course was rooted in shamanism, but in an eclectic and modern fashion. What Kennan has done since then is to extricate his Anglo-Celtic interests, explore them further and developed them into an outline. The themes in this course are a progression of all the material that has emerged in his journey around his heritage.

However, the core of this project involves him and his

journey, and remains partially obscure, even to Kennan, and maybe always will be. It centres around the idea of what the soul was considered to be in this Heathen period; how it informed all the other facets that he has explored, and are now outlined in the course he is developing – modern medicine included. He is excited that this Heathen concept of body and soul – as a unified complex – is the foundation of an authentic health and medical worldview that 'talked' not only at that period of time, but remains with us still.

I am sure there is more to tell here. But it is not yet clear, being researched and starting to be written. I am aware that Kennan is now deep in the realms of a magical worldview from which his creative imagination and fertile ideas will reveal more over time. He is not reluctant to express this process, being a wordsmith of his tradition and, in his words, a modern Anglo-Celtic Medicine Man.

I am now happy to close this chapter on the story and move into areas that I am sure will interest the modern reader. We can now move into and explore the place of modern medicine; medicine as an establishment, and the whole Medical Industrial Complex in more detail through the lens of Kennan's vision. We can then take a somewhat speculative step into seeing what the future of medicine holds; what the present transition is negotiating, and how the inevitable transformation may unfold.

Fifteen

I would like to return to Ian's input, but now beginning with my voice:

I notice, in the account to date, that my voice has diminished or, at least, changed. This is because Ian has used it directly as a voice for my stories, or otherwise quoted me, where he thinks appropriate. This is all interspaced with his account and reflections. Okay, that seems a useful and reasonable way to go about this business, but in so doing, I notice the stories have diminished and stopped altogether, and ask myself why or what that signifies?

I think the stories somehow set the stage for my career, so the ones at the beginning would have had a greater impact before I became familiar with medicine more generally. After this, similar issues would not so surprise me. However, I have noticed in my work that others come to the surface, and from all over the place in my story. I think this because they emerge in response to something someone has said or asked, and these can come from anywhere in my career.

As Ian and I progressed, my own story has come to the fore and predominated. So, the prior stories were the ones that had an impact on me in the telling of this account, and were not selected to appease an anticipated audience. In fact, I find it difficult to write for or perform in front of an unseen audience; I prefer feedback and interchange. Ian has performed this function, and is one reason why I couldn't have written this account on my own; it has required a dialogue rather than my more journalistic style when I write.

Ian has told me that he wonders whether I am epileptic. He bases this view on the symptoms I experienced during the year up until I left practice; as well as maybe a bit of reference to some patterns in my story, such as my speculation about childhood autism. I was, at first, surprised. But he has picked up other things in my account that have surprised me, such as the description of Ann's cancer as an orange, and then using the same metaphor for my liver abscess. I am also reminded that his medical interests were mainly in neurological medicine.

I am also aware that many practitioners of psychiatry, or other areas of psychological medicine, can tend to look at some mental disturbance in a neurological way, such as with attention deficit disorders, autism, and epilepsy. I think there may be at least two factors in this. One is a preference to not lapse into personality disorder diagnoses, which some (including I) cringe about. The second is the profound confusion that still exists in medicine between the brain and the mind, and their association.

I now notice that Ian has viewed me in both these lights. He has reflected a fair amount about ascribing me a personality diagnosis, particularly at the beginning of our meetings, but his neurological views are recent and not documented to date. Maybe he did not want his own subjective appreciation in this area to impinge on the account, but I am more than a little intrigued, because this approaches the field of shamanism, the anthropological study of which is littered with both these perspectives.

Without going into any detail about my symptoms of now nearly a decade ago, I am surprised I did not see them as epileptic at the time. I saw them more in the migraine category, after I had looked at all sorts of physiological pattern triggers, such as fluctuations in blood sugar and stress hormone levels, after excluding diagnoses like diabetes. Yet now I think about it, the episodes do have an epileptic quality. Because other issues intervened in that period, I did not undertake the sort of investigations, such as EEG (electroencephalogram) or an MRI that may have shed further light on them. And I am unlikely to do so now they have abated and disappeared.

The phenomenon of epilepsy is intriguing. Look at the use of ECT (electroconvulsive therapy) in depression. ECT was originally used because there was found to be an inverse relationship between schizophrenia and epilepsy, in that schizophrenics (generally under medical care) rarely had epilepsy. Then the logic went something like this: Induce epilepsy in schizophrenics and we cure their madness! Well, apart from the logic of this, and the ethics of applying such crazy reasoning to use it as a basis of a barbaric treatment, it is something that wouldn't happen today. But the outcome was even more strange, it didn't work for schizophrenics, but for those who also had an affective disorder – depression – it helped, and sometimes significantly.

Putting aside the incompatible fact that shamans are often seen as either schizophrenic and epileptic, or both, what does this tell us? Well, whilst I was a psychiatric registrar administering ECT, I thought I'd put the treatment to the test. During one period of personal depression, I locked the door, darkened my room, lay down, and did some cyclic breathing. I then consciously initiated a shaking in my feet, as I had witnessed during ECT, and allowed the shaking to progress up and through my body. Eventually the shaking kind of 'took over', and I allowed it to spontaneously to affect my whole body and then diminish altogether, of its own accord. And, afterwards, I felt much, much better emotionally for several days. I didn't, however, have any major insights or earth-shattering visions, bugger it, just the feeling of wellbeing that sometimes bordered on euphoria.

Then, in my eastern spiritual sojourns, I came across the idea of Kundalini energy, and the pennies started to drop. Without going into the specific mythological details of Kundalini, it is, in essence, the movement of physical energy through the body in a vibrating manner. The energy is considered to move up the spine from its base, to enter the head to result in bliss and spiritual enlightenment. The associations with ritual rhythmic dancing and such cultural phenomena as the Whirling Dervishes of Islam did not escape my notice. It is a short step to see this in the shamanic traditions, and considering shamans themselves as epileptic.

But was – am – I an epileptic? Do I use alcohol, in the manner of hallucinogens maybe, to 'loosen' the energy that is blocked? Because I certainly experience psychic states and sometimes visions with the use – conventional misuse – of alcohol. I certainly wondered about autism as a child, and I still have an autistic tendency in normal situations unless inspired, when I am able to use language and abstract concepts quite freely. In fact, this is now my norm, so I avoid situations that are mundane and unstimulating. I don't think I am epileptic in the conventional sense, maybe not even in the marginal category; but I do use epileptic patterns in my psychic economy, sometimes regularly.

Shamans are also given a frequent tar and feathering of personality disorder diagnoses, many of which I note Ian has attributed to me. Does this make me angry or concerned? No. Why? Well, in one sense I have got used to it and them, and they now wash off me. This concern was one reason I went into therapy in the first place. I feel I can see the 'other side' of such disorders; I can empathise with the pain of lack of feeling in the borderline personality, I understand the intent and power of the psychopath. But I see these as labels that describe the person but, ultimately, not who they are. And that includes me, too. If I get that from anyone these days, I show them the door.

Psychotic? Am I that? I get depressed, sometimes

profoundly. It was the core reason I went into therapy: I was depressed, had used one of my usual tricks – sex – to try and deal with it, but only to temporary relief (pun intended). Apart from the fact that the sex didn't remain just sex (I fell in love), it was the failure to be able to negotiate the depression on my own that led me to therapy. If I knew what I knew now, maybe I would have sought beyond a Jungian to a shaman, maybe with some good hallucinogens thrown in!

Some see me as a little crazy, even mad. I don't see that in myself; in fact, I am annoyed often by the effort it takes me to get into trance states and other altered states of consciousness. I could have lapsed more readily into plant-based hallucinogens – I would avoid chemical manufacture – were I not to have alcohol. It is part of my culture, I'm sure my forefathers used it liberally, although I now suspect it was often mixed up with the aforesaid plants. After all, alcohol is good for storage and preserving.

Shamans are often judged as being psychotic and specifically schizophrenic. With the aforementioned incompatibility with an epileptic diagnosis, I find this very interesting. It may be due to schizophrenics under clinical care not being florid, somehow stunted in their process, and often tranquillized. Maybe the two conditions do go together, and the epileptic is the neurological whilst psychosis the psychological manifestation. Maybe the problem, as ascertained by my own ad hoc researching, is that schizophrenics should indeed be induced into epilepsy, and vice versa. But maybe ECT is the wrong way of doing it. Sex, drugs, and rock and roll may indeed be the way!

I'm getting irreverent. I also don't know whether this has clarified anything at all in the reader's mind, except to add to the confusion. But it is confusing and more than a bit chaotic, that's the nature of the territory.

Now I'll hand the wheel back to Ian.

This is Ian, and I'm back at the wheel; a bit crook, but wanting to move forward.

We were now out of the woods and moving toward open territory with respect to Kennan's story; we are standing in the present. Before moving out into the open to gain some vision of a speculative future horizon, I feel it was time to take stock and ask him some general questions about the state of health of modern medicine, because I know he sees it to be in 'poor health'; but does this indicate that it is terminal?

Kennan doesn't believe we had arrived at that point as yet, although the turning point beyond which it may be considered terminal is usually only clarified and defined in hindsight. In this respect, the situation is a little like climate change, in that we don't as yet know whether we have passed a point of no return. However, he is adamant that we always have the capacity to change the course of healthcare and maybe reduce or even avert the need for a more apocalyptic changing process: A smoother transition if we take action sooner rather than later, it would seem, but a transition nonetheless.

Kennan is equally adamant that this involves medicine relinquishing some of the sacred cows of beliefs it is presently founded on, as well as much of its power and control. It is a bit of a paradox to our way of thinking: Modern medicine may need to give up some power and control to remain relevant and involved in the future of health; if it doesn't, then the sweeping changes may relegate it to history. He also believes that medicine needs to stop ignoring, denying, and even lying about many obvious questionable and dubious facts; although he sees this as a problem with science in general.

I wondered if he is being overly dramatic here with his metaphors and opinions, and then he surprises me. Kennan indicated that maybe that isn't the point. He suggests that, irrespective of whether we collectively believe that climate change is 'real' or not, is, in some ways, irrelevant; considering that it is real, and thus changing our ways makes for a more sustainable and healthy future anyway.

In this respect, Kennan sees an exact parallel to healthcare and medicine's position within it. Instead of taking a defensive and protectively aggressive stance towards such issues as environmental poisoning and vaccination, medicine needs to address the public concerns, openly and cooperatively, as well as look at the facts without coloured lenses. If he – Kennan – as an individual found this not to be difficult, then why couldn't the profession as a whole? Actually, this is a rhetorical question; he does understand why the profession can't, it just saddens and disappoints him.

After this preliminary discussion, it struck me we could just go around in circles with rational argument, so we needed a point of departure. The first was the premise that modern western medicine – MWM – is in trouble; so, what evidence could he voice for this?

Kennan was aware that it would be easy to outline the areas of difficulty and conflict. He had already hinted at vaccination, although not the specific public concerns regarding toxic additives in vaccines. He also points to other environmental areas of concern, such as water treatment, GMO foods and nutritional production generally. The pharmaceutical area is rife with concern, led by such drugs as statins for high cholesterol and mental health drugs generally. Then there is the avoidance of safe alternatives to drug treatment, particularly in the hormone and immune system areas. Is all the surgery we perform necessary? What of mental health? The list goes on …

Maybe we will cover some of these issues as Kennan's story progresses, but at this point he feels this is the wrong way to address the problems.

"Why?" I ask.

"Because it will get the profession's back up. They will hide behind so-called evidence-based medicine, not only because they might be seen to be wrong, but because they may have something to protect. There is a huge amount of vested interest in medicine and they are not going to give up control easily. It is better to try and increase the information generally; kind of flood the market with information so that politically, economically, and even scientifically the various institutions simply have to take note."

"You don't think that is happening already?" I counter.

"Yes," he agrees, "but it is still somewhat reactionary. One of the good things, believe it or not, is social media and Dr Google. Of course, there are lots of pitfalls with them in this arena of information, but they spearhead a movement that is increasingly demanding to be heard. It is simply that this movement could be better organised and more creative with what it wants to achieve and how it goes about it, which it will do over time."

"Well," I smile, "I know that is the nature of your vocation now, up to and including this story! So, inform me – us – how can this be addressed?"

Kennan explains that we need to get away from the restricted scientific area – for reasons we will come to – to try and get a broader picture, which both professionals and the public can relate to, because even the professionals struggle with the science. To do this, he chose four points that closely follow other observers in the field, who are also making similar comments and raising concerns.

The first was that the cost of healthcare was rising at an alarming and ultimately unsustainable rate. Kennan could outline the forces that contribute to this, but wants to focus on the emotional undercurrent that permeated all four points. He identifies this as fear, pure and simple: Fear of death, disease, pain, or infirmity – but ultimately fear. What does not help this, now that politics and business have effectively taken over medical funding, is that the public have an unreasonable belief that healthcare and medicine specifically should be freely available and free of charge.

The public are also voting with their feet, by accessing alternative and complementary healthcare products and their practitioners in increasing numbers. This is the second point, and closely allies with other issues in this section, where the emphasis is on things 'natural'. This is significant in many ways; for example, seeing modern medicine itself as somehow unnatural, that the relationship with doctors does not sustain the public in a social sense. This is in spite of the fact the most fees and product costs for alternative healthcare are from the family budget; this being somewhat ironic and a bit of a paradox when modern medicine is also expected to be free.

Thirdly, doctors are leaving in droves; dissatisfied, diseased, or dead. Kennan maintains that a significant part of this is that the selection process for medical school is based on academic criteria, and not the prior exposure to and acquaintance of the demands of being a doctor, as in the past: The 'apprenticeship' viewpoint. Kennan sees medical practice as an art, first and foremost, and that the interpersonal skills and capabilities of a prospective medical student are not taken into sufficient account. At the other end of the spectrum, doctors are leaving because they are stressed, tired and fed up. The incidence of mental health concerns and suicide is alarming. In this respect, Kennan's story is one account amongst many. I find it ludicrous that someone with his skills and experience is now potentially languishing.

Of most concern, and fourthly, is the phenomenon of the 'worried well'. We live longer than we ever have and also have this vast array of science and technology to support, treat, and care for us. Yet it is a paradox that, in spite of all this knowledge and expertise, we remain frightened about our health. Along with financial concerns, this keeps the insomniacs awake more than anything else. Why is this? Don't we fundamentally trust MWM?

"There is no simple answer," explains Kennan. "One of the problems is that, in spite of our supposedly advanced mental abilities, we tend to look at issues in a very cognitively restricted way. We have these following four points or issues in looking for them. We look for causes with diseases like cancer, when maybe there just isn't any. We break things down and dissect them in order to understand how they work, and maybe unwittingly kill the beast that we are looking for in so doing. We rely on quantities – statistics – for evidence, which is the incomplete basis of evidence-based medicine. We have an oppositional, or dualistic way of approaching problems; we see them as 'either-or', instead of 'both-and'.

"To fully understand and appreciate these four points, and the many others that support and overlap them, we need to look more broadly, particularly when the simplistic cognitive approach does not work. We are limited in thinking in an abstract way. For example, if the models for cancer we have are not providing solutions, how else can we reconceive it, imaginatively and creatively? We do not fully acknowledge the emotional and feeling dimensions: What does the fear signify, how do we look at it from both an individual and a collective perspective? Ultimately, these indicate a more holistic orientation; so maybe I should leave these four points hanging in the air as questions, whilst we start to look for some solutions."

To my way of thinking, Kennan is drawing attention to the problem of modern medicine in a different and more constructive way. I know I would take each of these four points and look at each in a kind of rhetorical way; questions that do not demand answers, instead raising more examination and further questions maybe. Because, whatever the solutions, we have yet to ask the right questions and look in the right direction. In Kennan's metaphoric words: "We have an elephant in the room!"

Kennan identifies a significant 'other' influence on the way he approaches MWM; that is, his spiritual inquiry. He did not undertake this inquiry in an attempt to deal with the conundrums he was experiencing in medicine, but as an inner imperative. This was what originally led him into Jungian analysis, although this somewhat inevitably threw him back into medicine. In fact, everywhere he inquired he came across a significant component around health, such that he started to see health and spirituality as inextricably linked, and that health itself is a legitimate pathway to spiritual development. Within himself, I note, he is rediscovering the principles and archetypal patterns of shamanism.

One effect of this enquiry is that Kennan began to see his personal life, and the culture in which it is embedded, in a greater and vaster perspective. It stretched well beyond his own personal existence into his ancestry, such that exploration of the whole Anglo-Celtic world held importance, meaning, and purpose for him. As he delved further, and using what he called the 'shamanic complex' as a guide, he unearthed the patterns of health and medicine that existed in this earlier ancestral time.

This Heathen perspective, that we covered in the last meeting with respect to Kennan's latter years away from medical practice, made him realise that the current medical system is very restricted and not the panacea to health and wellbeing that he had been given to believe in his training. MWM is built around the modern era and the domination of science and technology. Historically, it is a product of the Christian era, which itself is built on Mediterranean culture. In essence, it is not indigenous to the peoples of northern Europe as, say, herbal or even folk medicine is.

Added to this is the opening up of the world to other cultures and hence their health systems. We are accustomed to some that have even become mainstream, though not usually with the system they come with. Acupuncture is a good example here. It derives from Traditional Chinese Medicine, or TCM, which is now a significant component of complementary medicine, both in theory and practice. But TCM is not alone, there is Ayurvedic Medicine from India, and others.

There is a mixture of alternative medical systems from other cultures, and even deep within our own, knocking at the door that many people will be exposed to if they – as many are – venture to see an alternative or complementary practitioner, when MWM fails them. Instead of either treating these systems in a deprecatory manner, or subjecting their methods to restrictive western scientific analysis, MWM should be asking what it lacks that these systems offer and whether they work. But to do this, MWM would have to accept that the individual's story and their response is a fundamental, and not trivially dismiss it as merely anecdotal, as it tends to.

Kennan's inquiry goes further than simply adopting another alternative system; indeed, he hasn't yet unearthed the 'system' he would believe in, he feels! But it does bring some unusual rewards, such as the fact that we are not necessarily taller and with bigger brain capacity than we have been at other periods in history. And that cancer and heart attacks were a rarity even until a hundred or so years ago. Or that, beyond the ravages of childbirth, trauma and infection, people lived longer and healthier than we do now, with significantly less markings of the so-called diseases of civilisation and ageing, such as osteoarthritis.

Why did Hippocrates, the so-called father of modern medicine, eschew 'the knife' for tumours? And why has the emphasis on nutrition and herbs been ignored? What about the humoural theory of medicine that was present until the modern era, or the role of ritual – present in disguise with the taking of medications – not acknowledged and explored? Why do we not listen to our patients, when they unexpectedly heal from a disease, as to what they did, and inquire of their mindset and story? Why are we so frightened that we use terms like 'spontaneous remission' and 'incorrect initial diagnosis' on their file? And maybe most significantly, why have we not explored the placebo effect in depth and detail?

It seems to me that Kennan is a polymath, who brings his wide learning and knowledge to bear on a discipline that tends to be restricted and does not engage other influential and relevant disciplines. As Kennan is at pains to point out, health is integral to our very being, personally and spiritually. It demands such a wide perspective and that itself is one reason why MWM is in the difficulty it is. Kennan is also a polemicist, and loves to debate and argue his position. That he has the confidence born of belief to do this, should not be forgotten.

Kennan does not see the modern western perspective of medicine as the end point, or necessarily directed toward it. He believes medicine will continue to evolve and change, maybe quite significantly in the current era; but what he would like to see is that MWM retains an important and valuable place in this change. If it resists, this is where he sees a more apocalyptic scenario emerging. But, as discussed earlier, he believes we have the opportunity to both create and change the future. First and foremost is MWM recognising its limitations and weaknesses, and looking beyond its own parameters, when what it is presently doing is patently not working.

Kennan explains that there were many metaphoric visual

lenses we could use to look at the problem that is MWM. What he had done is simply choose a way of looking at it that suits his temperament, but which he believes has a wider application. I must admit that I now appreciate his way to look at the problem; it has given me a line of inquiry outside of my habitual custom; after all, I had been indirectly 'taught' by MWM, and further to see its approach as the only way of looking at medicine. Similarly, to provide a brief overview of the depth of history and culture within which MWM is placed has given me an expanded perspective, which makes me look at areas like complementary medicine and even new age healing modalities in a different light.

The issue of restoration of depth implies we are lacking this in our present western culture, I surmised: Was this Kennan's opinion as well?

"Yes." The reply was unequivocal. "I am not the only person to comment on this, and I do like one word that describes our current worldview: Flatland. We have a kind of two-dimensional view of the world and our place in in, and ignore the further operative dimension of depth. This depth leads us into the disciplines I have outlined, but also others like anthropology, archaeology, mythology, history, and many others, all of which have a health component, if you look for it. However, these are beyond my capacity to integrate beyond a point. Rather, I would like to give some further viewpoints and mental models to help build the overall thrust of my argument."

The flatland perspective means we live a restricted existence, argues Kennan. One outcome of this is we lose the depth and wisdom of a spiritual worldview, when even religion has become flattened and somewhat irrelevant in the West, at least to and in medicine. This leads to many distortions, such as a view of life as a linear process ending in extinction, or death, which we then existentially fear.

Accordingly, medicine becomes directed to postponing death

under the illusion, or more appropriately the delusion, that somehow it will go away if we do this long enough. Kennan points to the way we deal with death in the elderly as an example, as well as the intense focus on pathological process in the body, which we both fear and are attracted to at the same time. As an illustration, he points out how family, friends, and even strangers are attracted to someone in the community who develops terminal cancer, particularly if this is a child or young adult.

This amounts to a view in our culture that the pinnacle of life is somewhere between 21 and 28 years of age, and that life is apparently all downhill after this point. Kennan indicates the many cultural and social issues that point to this, both in our society at large with the unrealistic desire to recapture our youth, and a medicine that uses parameters of a twenty-odd year-old when examining an older person. Added to this is the pursuit of wealth, with the illusion that it will lead to happiness, security, or whatever psychological deficiency it is that fuels the chase in the first place.

A way of understanding why we are so literally bound to our earthly existence is a fault of both medicine and religion. If we are not exposed to and appreciate the wisdom and mystery of birth, sex, and death, then we lack the initiatory changes and maturation such exposure garnishes. Birth and death are too often associated with hospitals and taken out from sight, when in the past they were more socially and communally integrated.

Previously this was the domain of religion, which would still seem to have a mortgage on sex; except medicine is getting its claws in here too, with the fear of the consequences of sex bound up with infection and disease. It seems that modern religion has passed its obligation over these domains to the medical profession who, in their turn, have pathologised them, or socially removed them with all sorts of social and psychological ramifications and consequences, particularly as agencies of initiation.

What Kennan is pointing out here is the role of ritual in our lives as a function of rites of passage, maturity and wisdom. Ritual is also a component in the shamanic complex. But why the shamanic complex? Because, he maintains it is as deep as one can go in the exploration of health, healing and medicine. It contains the primordial patterns – the so-called complex in Kennan's terms – that govern our earthly existence and includes our health within this. In Jung's terms this is archetypal, or the prototype, stereotype, or primal pattern to which we should refer.

In the discipline of philosophy, this pattern of depth is called the perennial philosophy. In this model, a continuum is drawn that extends from the body to the mind, emotions and ultimately spirit. This is also a model that permeates eastern spirituality and has healing reflected within it, as in the chakra system. This philosophy, or the great chain of being of birth, sex and death can be varied, added to, or adjusted to suit cultural viewpoints. But the fundamental pattern remains the same. It describes the inner life of man and his place in the universe. It also is a very good descriptor for mental distress, but that's another story...

Or is it? In fact, the great chain of being is a model that is employed in the modern era within the holistic health movement. So, it is no great surprise that alternative health employs eastern models that inherently contain them, and to great effect. However, Kennan is adamant that we are western and have such models in our own heritage; we just need to dig a little deeper and look for them, because they may suit our temperament – our psychic 'DNA' – more suitably.

As a slight detour, Kennan used the great chain of being model as an example of how we could reconceive mental distress, by seeing it as an imbalance. He highlighted that each of the levels – physical, mental, emotional and spiritual – was progressively included in the next level up, but that this higher level was greater than its predecessor; a bit like Russian dolls. In this view then physical disorder and emotional distress will have an indirect and effect on mental stability, which we may not countenance and look for. In reverse, a spiritual view completely includes the mental, and more, which raises some interesting implications.

However, Kennan is keen to leave elaboration here until we approach the future of medicine argument, instead pointing out that this model provides a strong position in any genuine holistic health and medical model. But he is at pains to further point out that this is just one half of the story, because it tends to highlight the 'inner' world at the expense of external reality; a fault of adopting an exclusively eastern approach, in his opinion. As Kennan describes it, there is the reflection of this model in the world, which must take account of the familial, social, occupational and environmental domains. These could be varied and elaborated on, but yet again, the principle holds valid. In Kennan's worldview, these two models come together at the body, at one end, and in spirit, at the other. In his opinion, this is how extensive and inclusive holism is, and this is also inclusive of health, by definition.

It is this model Kennan has been working on in the last three years, with its application to health and medicine generally. He sees it as particularly relevant to the concern of mental health in the West, and is seriously concerned that we adopt this greater perspective rather than the simplistic, mechanical and biological one that we presently use. In fact, his concern about the way we look at mental health is for the future not only of medicine, but also for western culture.

I am aware we will be exploring these themes more as we move further into the future, but I would not want to diminish their significance simply because we have skated over a vast lake.

I am beginning to appreciate, at the level of MWM at least, that unless we can appreciate and understand mental healthcare in a different light than we currently do, then we are in serious difficulty. Not only because of how we currently manage mental distress, but because it is such a significant and integral component of all physical health that confronts the medical practitioner.

I am also increasingly aware that medicine has become dominated by the scientific worldview. Although Kennan has drawn frequent attention to this, specifically with relation to the role of religion and the ignored position of spirituality – the two are fundamentally different as I am sure he will explain – I was still a little unclear about it. I also realise that would be where his argument would head next.

"You used the term 'scientism' a little earlier. Could you elaborate on this?" Although I was leading the discussion with this question, I had little doubt that this would initiate the next stage in this process.

"Okay, that's a good lead in to where I would like to go next, so let's kick off there."

I drew a small sigh of relief. However, it was inevitable according to Kennan, and I was now also experiencing that our discussions attain this psychic synchrony. I settled down to listen to his views about science and its role in health and medicine.

Kennan called science 'scientism' for a particular reason, although he was not alone in the use of that term. He saw that in the modern era science had usurped much of the ground previously held by religion. There was a reason for this: Religion was no longer satisfying the individual spiritual urge, and in the Age of Enlightenment, science seemed a ready successor. The problem with this is that we are under the illusion that evolution is synonymous with progression, and that science has superseded religion as some sort of advancement. Human hubris runs deep.

However, science is failing in this task, as it inevitably will, in Kennan's opinion. Were it to be succeeding, then healthcare – a ready arbiter of spiritual wellbeing and the religion that should contain it – would be healthy itself. Patently it is not, and it is no accident that alternative and complementary healthcare with a strong spiritual component should be filling the void. In Kennan's opinion, science has become a pseudo-religion called scientism, which is already failing us. Should there be doubt around this view, he suggests – once again – that we reflect on the mess that climate change is in.

And, as Kennan points out, if we doubt that health is connected to spirituality in this way, then we are denying our own religious heritage. Because Jesus was not only responsible for physical healing, such as the blind seeing and the lame walking, he was also involved in mental health, by casting out demons. As an aside, exorcism is a very shamanic practice. Yet Jesus was also able to bring the dead back to life, and is something that he was able to do himself. In fact, the shamanic elements predominate in the life of Jesus.

How does modern medicine compare? Not well, it would seem. Should a miracle occur, such as someone surviving a life-threatening disease or death sentence, we question the diagnosis, or see it as something like spontaneous remission. We do not explore the stories of such people and their seemingly miraculous cures; we would do well to do so. Many have noted the relationship with mental health here but, again, this is poorly explored. What is the significance of the placebo effect? And why does hypnosis work? Why do people suffer differently from an identical disease or injury? The list goes on … But back to science, and specifically the pharmaceutical management of illness and disease. I note reluctance in Kennan to approach this subject:

"It's vast and many are doing it. Maybe I should just give some pointers from my perspective?" A rhetorical question: He was going to proceed anyway.

"Pharmacy, if I can use that general term, is basically derived from a religious background, and a more natural and magical one at that." Kennan went on to outline pharmacy's relationship to nature, generally, and the herbal kingdom, in particular. Pharmacy is actually built on herbal medicine, with the addition of chemistry, commonly associated with the alchemist-physician Paracelsus. From this point on – the late 16th century – medical treatment took an increasingly chemical outlook, divorcing itself from its mystical roots in alchemy, as religion itself lost precedence in health and healing to scientific rationalism. Paracelsus would not approve.

Kennan held to the spiritual view that nature provides for us, even to the maxim that there is a herb for every health condition. He believes that modern pharmacy is built on the arrogance that we can improve upon nature, aided and abetted by the other issues that have become associated with pharmacy, and thus developing it into an industry, big business.

Yet he sees vestiges of the magic that is associated with herbs and the healer. The pattern of use of pharmaceutical medication is an unwitting acknowledgement of the power of ritual. However, he is concerned about Wordsworth's injunction that "we murder to dissect", in that something is inextricably lost in the relentless and seemingly endless process of drug improvement.

One of the ironies is that, even with the best motives, pharmaceutical medications are foreign to the body; technically they are poisons, all of them. They are ceasing to work therapeutically; that is, if they ever did according to the manufacturer's claims. They are also increasingly expensive and create an unhealthy dependency on the medical profession, and in turn on the pharmaceutical industry. Addiction has many levels.

One further point Kennan elucidated was that more drugs than we realised had mental consequences, such as blood pressure and cholesterol-lowering medications. He reiterated that the mind and the brain are not the same thing: The brain is an organ of the body, connected to the mind that extends far beyond it; rather like the television is connected to channels in the air. Medications alter the television, not the channels, and this includes both the lack of specificity of medications used for treating bodily illness, as well as those specifically used for mental distress.

Technology itself is another product of science and hence the potential victim of scientism. The extraordinary advances that we have, rather like antibiotic resistance because of overuse, are coming back to bite us. Increasingly expensive and insatiable with its promise to cure us of all illness, including death, the public now see it as a panacea. The only problem is that it is not living up to expectations. This is partly because the medical premise of disease is that it is built on causes. What this means is that we look for one, but in failing to find it assume that there is still one hiding there, and we just need further advances to find it and utilise this knowledge in our favour.

One example of this is early detection. We assume that cancer is caused by a mutation that then gets out of control, so that the earlier we find it, then the greater the chance of cure. This is not proving the case; in fact, it is getting us into more of a medical tangle and engaging other agencies, like the legal profession. In Kennan's opinion, the model we have of such diseases is wrong and a cure will never eventuate on such terms.

But what does a cure mean? In simple terms, it means that a disease is eradicated, permanently. If it returns, then it is assumed the treatment has failed, when it may be that the circumstances that allowed the disease to manifest are still present and operative. Also, even when pronounced cured, a patient will still worry about the disease returning and the incessant medical check-ups belie the confidence that all is permanently well.

In Kennan's opinion, we need to resurrect the term healing, itself related to the word whole, and hence holism. Healing is different from curing: Healing is making whole, plus or minus the illness or disease that made the recipient un-whole in the first place. In this view, we can be healed and still die: At a spiritual level, this is the acceptance that whatever we are afflicted with us is to take us to our graves – and maybe beyond.

And with the term heal we need to revisit the title healer and his or her relationship to magic. Because doctors are presently unwitting magicians; poorly trained in that art as they are generally not apprentices and initiates, and therefore lacking insight into the power they have at their disposal to wield.

"Let's draw a line in the sand here, Ian, there's much more we could explore. But I think we should leave this as some sort of testament to how I see medicine in the present era moving forward. There are multitudes of stories and examples I could use to back the arguments and embellish the discussion, but maybe that is for another setting."

I believed him to be referring again to his preference for other settings for this disclosure.

Sixteen

I have decided to provide the reader a summary of Kennan's views of medicine in the next two chapters. As the narrative to date has provided a progressive, cyclic, sometimes meandering and maturing perspective, I thought it might help for me to integrate this into some sort of cohesive whole. I feel that not only will it be a useful resource for the reader to refer to, but it will also help me professionally. I will do this by using the present chapter to cover the more general issues concerning and confronting medicine that we have covered in Kennan's narrative to date, and the next chapter to focus on specific health issues; that is, illnesses and diseases as we currently view them.

I would like to point out that the views and opinions in the next two chapters are those of Kennan, and presented by me in an integrated and summary form; they are not necessarily my own. Even though he will not feature again until the final chapter, Kennan has read and endorsed my words. He, like me, feels that sometimes he needs a translator of sorts! Having said this, I must admit that Kennan's views have provided a deeper context for my own experience and increasingly represent my own position as well, such that I imagine my position may ultimately mirror his.

The reader may wonder how much the trauma in Kennan's life, most particularly of a few years ago with respect to leaving medicine, has coloured his insights and conclusions; indeed, this is a question I had to ask myself. Has he been wounded? Yes. But life is about wounding and healing, he may well argue. So, is he healed? Since his pneumonia encounter, I would say yes, although he remains scarred. Yet he sees those scars now to be of wisdom; if they itch, he scratches them and something is revealed. Kennan's view of his past is realistic; he sees the personal agendas and games that people play, and the fears that drive them. Those that have been played out to his detriment he accepts, but doesn't have to like. I would still suggest that those who fall in this latter category cross the road should they encounter him; his strong eye is enough for most.

There are two major themes that stand out for me, because grasping their significance makes an understanding and appreciation of other themes much more available. The first is that Kennan reverses our usual reality perspective of trusting the physical senses and consensus reality as the primary position in health; indeed, of life as a whole. He does not deny its place and importance but sees that it is commonly restricted to what he refers to as the mechanical worldview from which all other phenomena – and most particularly those that lie outside this worldview – are commonly viewed. In medicine, he sees this position to view all metaphysical concerns, such as the non-biomechanical mind, as a product or consequence of the physical or biomechanical.

Kennan sees things the other way around. He understands that our physical reality is somehow embedded in, and dependent on, a far greater, non-physical, and ultimately mysterious reality. This inevitably restricts our health ministrations, but it also makes them realistic and doesn't pretend that we will one day be able to reduce the non-physical, or metaphysical ('beyond the physical'), into the physical. Instead, we respect the metaphysical and work in cooperation with it. This has enormous implications for the way we manage death, as well as diseases such as cancer.

The second theme is his respect for tradition and our need to remain in connection with its accumulated wisdom. Kennan sees science, specifically, to have lost this connection. In tradition, he sees the full picture of a phenomenon like health in what he calls an archetypal or holistic perspective. And, further, that unless we have that archetypal perspective of health, medicine will inevitably be incomplete and limited in range and effect.

However, Kennan does not see this as a flight into the past. He uses metaphors: Sometimes a dammed river needs to find other tributaries to negotiate the blockage; or, we may need to first go back to be able to go forward. These metaphors indicate both his preference for process over structure, as well as providing a more cyclic rather than a linear worldview. As an aside, he believes that a cyclic or spiral perspective provides connections to the metaphysical reality, which a linear one does not. It is also distinctive in that he sees the mind as primarily metaphysical and not as a by-product of the physical, specifically the brain; the position held by most neuroscience and psychiatry.

At various points in the narrative, Kennan has drawn a comparison to the views of quantum physics as a way of explaining his experience. Whilst premature, he does anticipate that a quantum view of reality will increasingly permeate our culture and help to transform science from a reductive technology to a creative art. Only by drawing on a quantum worldview, when confronted with the depths around his own illness and that of Ann, has he been able to intuitively grasp a greater health perspective that informs medicine far better, in his opinion. At a personal level, I know he credits it with the experiences that led to his loss of fear of death.

Of course, on their own, these two themes do not amount to a new paradigm of health and medicine, but they do point the way, I think. There are many other overlapping ideas that can come out of or be assembled in these two, but I am going to use them as a kind of window into a more holistic and archetypal perspective of health, which I am now convinced will ultimately lead to a changing of the paradigm itself.

Why do I think this? Because I understand that archetypal forces are powerful, and when we lose touch with them – as it can be argued modern medicine has – they will re-emerge. We also recognise their loss and look for them, sometimes elsewhere. In medicine, this is being seen in the alternative fields and now impacting on medicine itself. Kennan, it would seem, is a kind of voice or prophet of this re-emergence and the changes that result.

As an example, I would refer to the common catch-cry that we rue the loss of the old-fashioned doctor; the one who knew us, our families, and our trials and tribulations, and who was able to put any illness and disease into this wider context. We remember him or her with an emotional fondness and grieving that is not relieved by the efficiencies and expertise of the modern medical centre and its doctors.

This is a reference back to tradition, in Kennan's opinion. It was when the doctor was embedded in the broader social, familial and occupational dimensions of patient and family. He or she was more implicitly holistic in orientation; that is, carried more archetypal features of the healer. No wonder we long for this and bemoan its absence. There were non-tangible elements of healing present that no evidence-based medicine will ever discover. This longing is a reconnection, driven by emotion. Yet it is not a regression to a lost past, but to the images and feelings that are necessary for inclusion in the present and into the future.

Whilst this seems to be an example of the second theme outlined above, it also contains the first. Intuitively, because the doctor of old came from the broader holistic perspective that would even include his or her knowledge of the patient's mental and emotional states, he or she would diagnose and treat with respect for this greater perspective. So, both themes are covered;

tradition takes us back to a more holistic management that is metaphysical before it is physical. Tradition has recovered this more archetypal perspective and it is up to us to restore it in the present; a task in itself, but essential unless medicine loses its relevance at this basic practitioner level.

The fundamental orientation and principle of mind before matter – 'mind over matter' – has other broader implications. Inasmuch as science is directed toward matter, art is more the province of mind. Medicine, after all, is commonly or historically referred to as an art, The Art of Medicine. Have we forgotten so quickly?

The art of medical practice itself leads to all sorts of consequences. The doctor needs to listen to his or her patient, prior to examining them, and certainly before ordering investigations. Listening itself is an art, a bit of a lost one in the modern era; listening to a patient long enough will elicit not only their story but also what ails them and even guidelines to its management. This necessitates personal engagement with the patient; interpersonal connection; stepping into their reality. It requires the challenges of intimacy, and even eroticism, but it cannot be foregone.

Depersonalise medicine and the problem may be treated, even cured, but the patient will not be healed. The increasing dependence on technology and its brilliance cannot avoid the brute fact that the doctor is dealing with a living, breathing human being who feels and experiences fear of their malaise. Unless we engage with the heart as well as the head, all our efforts will be in vain. In only mechanically dealing with a problem, all we do is postpone it; because the factors that brought about its manifestation have not been elucidated and dealt with.

Instead of an inquiry that focuses on the presenting symptom and goes down the rabbit hole chasing a diagnosis, and hence a cause to be dealt with, we should be adopting a different approach. Rather like taking the broader view of mind that includes the body, we should make our inquiry similarly broad and watch the symptom emerge from it. Go back prior: When were things last okay? When did this change? How? Even further back: The family setting, the family's origins. Genetics devoid of its psychic correlation is similarly brute and mechanical.

This all amounts to a reversal of the normal medical inquiry. It takes time ... and expertise. It can be taught, but it demands apprenticeship and not a computer programme. As Kennan is quick to point out, we run into difficulties the minute we narrow our focus on diagnosis. Gnosis means 'knowledge' and 'dia-' can mean 'through'; that is 'through' the patient and their symptoms. However, 'dia-' can also mean 'apart'; that is, apart from the patient and in the hands of the doctor. It is Kennan's contention that we no longer see diagnosis as through, but apart and excluding the patient. Diagnosis can depersonalise, but also make the focus restricted to the point that we miss other relevant information. It also implies a solution; we think if we make a diagnosis, then there is something definitive we can treat and cure.

But such treatment is limited, as it is depersonalised. It fails to take the potentially omitted factors and other dimensions into account. And what if the diagnosis is wrong, as so often it is under these circumstances? Then we are committed to a treatment that may not only *not* be in our best interests as patients, but we will have to reverse the consequences of the resulting incorrect treatment as well, particularly if it is pharmaceutical, as it commonly is. And, if surgical, it is often completely irreversible. If the treatment doesn't work, dear doctor, maybe the diagnosis is wrong and the patient is not resistant, non-compliant, or 'idiosyncratic' in their response!

Kennan points out that the concept of syndrome is important, not only as an adjunct to any diagnosis, but as an ongoing way of looking at and managing any problem. By contrast, syndrome means 'moving together'; it is the opposite of 'apart' and implies a process with 'moving'. Syndrome collects the features the patient presents with and formulates them into some sort of flexible cohesion, able to be adjusted with new facts or elimination of wrong ones. Syndrome can include the non-physical comfortably and in a non-threatening manner to the practitioner.

All this reinstates the importance of the general practitioner, or GP. He or she is not a branded 'family doctor' (what a misnomer in modernity), but general in a holistic way. It is this that we see in the image of the so-called old-fashioned doctor. The GP is not competing with specialist medicine, as generalisation is a speciality in its own right; it is pointing to holism, after all.

What I would like to do now is select some issues about modern health, medicine and its management, which pertain to us all in a general way. I am going to look at these through Kennan's eyes, using the various metaphoric lenses of the themes above, plus the various discussions he and I have had about the topics to be discussed.

We both have serious concerns about the role of investigations in medicine. Not only do they depersonalise any problem, but they are also being used and even relied on for diagnosis, and so they can dictate management. They are also the basis for much in the way of evidence, and hence the cornerstone of evidence-based medicine that dictates protocols back to the doctor, so eliminating an individualised management approach, or contract between doctor and patient.

There is even much in the science itself that is open to

question. A varying number of pathology results will fall outside the normal range even with no disease, because this is statistically normal. Also, the bar of normality may be set incorrectly. It is uncommon to see kidney testing come back as abnormal, but I defy most in the west to have a normal cholesterol profile! Investigations are very useful to support or confirm a diagnosis or syndrome, and to monitor management, but too often we confuse the two.

What are we actually detecting with our increasingly subtle – and invasive – radiology? Are we misinterpreting what is normal here and with biopsies and histopathology generally because of this subtlety? Are we over-diagnosing because that is the brief of medicine, to detect pathology? Are we detecting physiological processes and interpreting them as pathological, because that is how we are trained?

This overlaps the area of so-called early detection. I know Kennan has serious concerns about early detection, believing that in many cases we might be misinterpreting a natural healing process and judging it to be pathological. This concern extends to cancer, specifically genital, breast, and skin cancers in my view, although Kennan extends it to a general principle. The issue is, we just don't know any more because we are discovering and treating things without knowing their cyclic or natural development over time, devoid of intervention.

This is a difficult area and I am not minimising what can be achieved. I just believe we need to take a step back and not be as driven as we are by fear, public pressure, corporate avarice and the like. Genetic research is a case in point, where the science has outstripped the ethics. Kennan, like I, doubts whether we are mature enough as a species to fully appreciate the implications and consequences of all we are unearthing. This is where the guiding principles of tradition and archetypal patterns are of great assistance.

In general, we would do well to pay more heed to nature than we do. To believe we can either dismiss or disrespectfully improve on nature and healing is a disturbing and vast arrogance. The pharmaceutical industry illustrates this problem; although here I want to focus on the science of pharmacy and its relation to health management, and not engage the politics or corporate concerns.

Pharmacy has two strands traditionally. The first stems clearly from nature and is the natural medicine of foods and herbs, such that the latter is an art and science in its own right. The second is the more recent foray of mankind into the retrieval of metals and other boons of nature for their use in industry as well as health. Traditionally, this was called alchemy; itself often considered the precursor of modern chemistry and pharmacy.

The pharmaceutical industry has made immense strides in these areas, detecting and utilising what it has learned and derived in a myriad of therapeutic ways. However, and this is a key point, in Kennan's opinion all these developments and improvements need to remain connected to their sources. If they become disconnected they become increasingly alien to the body, so that in treating any disease with pharmacy one also has to treat the consequences of the treatment as well.

That they have become disconnected, there is no doubt. Hence the general and increasing public movement back to nutritional and herbal medicine, as well as other health models that do not have these inherent difficulties. It is as if this is an instinctive and intuitive backlash in the public, that is being dealt with in a patriarchal and judgmental manner by the establishment, simply based on the fact that science is the supposed ultimate authority. There is a strong power dynamic operating here.

We have a vast armoury that we have developed from these primary sources of nature and its gifts; we just need to be circumspect. This means reserving their use for critical occasions and selectively in areas like palliative care. Routine use to quell symptoms of inevitable life challenges, such as a cold, do not require such intervention. All that happens is that we influence the immune system in an unpredictable manner and we have not as yet determined the consequences of this. A similar argument could apply to vaccination, but I will pass by this rabbit hole in the present context; we will return to it.

Giving such medication to our children may have unforeseen consequences, but it also teaches them we have a chemical for every ill. This becomes even more concerning in mental territory and is the genesis of much in the way of addictive patterning. Giving such medication in the anticipation of a disease outcome (for example; high blood pressure or cholesterol) is conceptually a very flawed argument; it is catering to fear, suiting vested interests, when there are almost invariably non-pharmaceutical alternatives. We can be lazy, it seems.

There are wider implications. We use chemicals routinely in our houses, in our bathrooms, and on our bodies. Industrial poisoning may be implicated in climate change, but we may kill ourselves with cosmetic and narcissistic kindness before this becomes a concern. Yet it does not stop there: What about the way we treat foods? All the additives, colourings, preservatives, flavourings and the like that we add. The substitution of refined sugar (a drug) for fat (a healthy part of our diet); I could go on. Suffice it to say, none of this was part of Kennan's medical training.

What then is modern western medicine good for? If I take the comments regarding pharmaceuticals immediately above, it is clear that there is potentially much that it is useful for and uniquely good at. So, what is the problem? The problem is that modern medicine does not know its boundaries, driven by a science that believes its achievements and scope are unlimited. Science has stepped into the realm of religion in so doing, hence Kennan's preference for the term 'scientism'. He also points out that medicine's default position is pathology and not physiology, as well as seeing its domain as the restricted material, physical, or biomechanical dimension of life, instead of all of it.

If we keep to the limited physical and pathological boundaries, then we have much that is good. Our accident and emergency medicine – even if 'fed' by our western lifestyle – is second to none. We can save babies, children, and adults in the face of inevitable death. What we may not be so good in determining is whether saving is the right thing to do in all cases. Ethics is, as yet, not part of medical training. The Hippocratic oath is not generally taken by graduating doctors either; Kennan did not, and I doubt if most have even read it.

The more I write, the more I realise it is the boundaries of modern medicine that is the problem rather than what medicine practices. In the right context, and for the right reasons, modern medicine has so much brilliance that we should stand in awe and honour it. It is just that it has outstripped its brief. And maybe this is not so much the fault of medicine, but the vacuum left by religion; the pressures from other political and economic quarters, as well as the demands of a seeming insatiable and fearful public.

Yet we have taken a journey, through Kennan's eyes, that has explored many of the reasons behind the difficulties that modern medicine finds itself it. So how can any change be successfully put into effect? The main problem is that it involves trauma, and the paradox is that pain and suffering is what medicine is charged to mitigate, so how do we cut this Gordian knot?

My understanding is that trauma itself is at the centre of this knot. Kennan has indicated, on many occasions, that it is the exploration of trauma that might resolve the issue, so I will follow his reasoning here. But there is a preliminary: All his research on the dynamics of ordered systems comes to the conclusion that there is a point when internal turbulence leads to inevitable change, or a revolution. In modern parlance we use terms like paradigm shift for this process, but the issue is, how much turbulence – or trauma – is essential and necessary for this to be both creative and successful?

Kennan's opinion is that to minimise the trauma in and of modern medicine, beyond what is necessary, two factors need to be appreciated; that increased awareness is vitally important, and that the change will come from the public and not the health professions. Maybe this is the – his – fundamental reason for this account becoming public.

We live in an accelerating society, so it seems. That, in itself, portends much change on the horizon, and is not simply confined to western medicine and healthcare. In fact, the changes may be so total that medicine will get dragged along kicking and screaming. However, I know that Kennan does not believe that scenario; he is of the opinion that changes in health can spearhead other change elsewhere; such is shamanic wisdom.

Kennan's reasoning for this is that health is so axiomatically total and pervasive, that if we can grasp the changes that medicine needs to undergo and metaphorically birth it into a new paradigm, then other cultural features will follow suit. In qualifying this, he points to tradition, indicating that the myth of Jesus was built around a revolutionary spiritual perspective that had healing interwoven in it. He also remarks that this is a feature of many spiritual revolutionaries, that health and social welfare are often distinguishing features.

This is a grand vision, and I am not sure I can fully subscribe to it, but I will keep an open mind. I do understand, though, that all the social, economic, and political signs point to significant change on the horizon. I have also noticed the accelerated change that I have experienced within the profession, but how can I grasp a further understanding of this, and how may the reader do likewise?

Kennan begins with stress. Not a strong feature of his medical training, stress has increased dramatically in importance and significance. Many physical diseases previously put down to other organic factors are now seen to be stress initiated, from heart disease to cancer. We now understand the mechanisms of stress much more deeply, from the body to the brain, and then the mind. We have the ability to intervene at various physical, emotional and mental levels to manage stress more adequately and efficiently.

We also appreciate its importance in our welfare. We are hardwired to manage a reasonable amount of stress. Too little or too much and we can become ill and can die. There are definable evolutionary and physiological reasons for all this, and we understand these in ever more detail. But still the stress of modern living rises and rises …

Now we are dealing with and understanding trauma more; not only as a consequence of stress (or, more correctly, our failure to properly deal with it), but also when afflicted on us unbeknownst. Trauma and stress are profoundly intertwined; as we understand one, we understand the other. Yet trauma is, in Kennan's opinion, the weaker partner and has not yet caught up in our intellectual understanding or methods of managing it. There is much work yet to be done.

Yet stress and trauma mirror our acceleration as a culture. They are the health markers to keep an eye on, more so than their disease consequences. Trauma, in particular, is at the forefront of our minds, whereas disease lags behind as a marker of change. Trauma is what Kennan has decided to focus on. Is this because it has marked his own life, or because his own life is a metaphor for the wider changes we are discussing and anticipating? Maybe it is both.

I would have thought that this exploration would take a psychiatric or even psychological orientation, were I to have explored it. But I have come to know Kennan well by now, and know that he eschews both. The reasons for this might have become apparent in the account to date, but I am acutely aware that he sees psychiatry as a failed speciality and that it will be confined to history, along with research and academic psychology. Rather, he takes a view of both that demands depth, such as occurred in the twentieth century with Freud and later Jung, and one that is outside of the clinical arena altogether.

Kennan is maybe a purist. He sees 'psyche' as referring to soul in an authentic manner, and that any true psychology is better in the spiritual than the academic or medical ranks. In the past, this was conventional religion, but now it is a more fundamental and eclectic spirituality that has yet maybe to show its full face to the world. He also sees psyche in this spiritual sense as the true field on which trauma is encountered.

In such a psychospiritual worldview trauma can be redefined. In fact, trauma may be the modern word for the religious suffering of old. Kennan now sees that trauma is the greater component of stress, and that it is unavoidable. And, at a spiritual level, trauma should not be avoided, but faced when so demanded. I know he sees trauma to be intimately wound up with our life's journey and overlapping such new age wordings as karma and fate, or destiny. Nor does he see this as necessarily confined to one's individual life, but bound up in a sense of ancestry and heritage that we may interpret as genetics, at some mundane level, or generational.

Kennan has often remarked that when he would see a patient

in practice with a disease of some standing, he could often recognise that this stemmed from a choice in the past when maybe the option appropriate to his patient was not taken. It was the line of so-called least resistance, supported by our modern culture maybe, but not the one the patient was being – spiritually – directed toward.

Obviously, such interpretations are idiosyncratic and easily available to criticism, but Kennan remains convinced of their validity born of his own experience; and, the more his spiritual insight developed, the more he could see these patterns. It has also given him the opportunity to assist people differently with their trauma in the present, knowing the potential consequences, although in practice such an orientation remains controversial and difficult to enact.

In a core way, I suspect it was this divergence from mainstream that stressed and ultimately traumatised the healer himself; prone and attracted as he was, with the choice of relationships such as Ann. In this, he is very much in the company of the shamans of old. I am not surprised he chose this path when the opportunity presented itself.

It is this fundamental variance – that such dynamics cannot be included in the current medical mainstream – that led to his departure, in my view. Yet he also sees that it is because mainstream cannot entertain such deeper views that it may well be doomed as a profession, and that these views will visit themselves on the health professions until they change, if they can. There are many signs of this in the personnel and philosophies of complementary and alternative medicine; it is just not yet in the mainstream.

When – not if – it does finally affect the mainstream will the turbulence then begin, if it is not happening already? Kennan's account of his psychiatric experiences shows such early signs over a generation ago. Then the seeds of renewal will need to emerge from the depths with those brave enough to champion them. There have been many who have done so to this point in time, but there is more work to be done.

What does all this mean for the individual? At a very practical level, it means learning ways to handle stress; not to get rid of it, but how to negotiate it. Living is inevitably stressful. What we need to do is accept this brute fact, not avoid it, but develop abilities – both psychological and physical – to deal with it. Although this all sounds simple, it is, in fact, something that requires education, support, and guidance.

Traumatic events will visit us; they are part of life. Of course, trauma comes in all shapes and sizes, sudden and slow-burning. But if we can handle the stress entailed in the process then we can start to look more deeply at the trauma and its relative wisdom: What is it telling us about our life? Our direction? Is it visiting us because we are going down the wrong road? Is it challenging us with something deeper about our individual destiny that we need to fulfil?

I know Kennan finds western views on trauma quite pathetic in their ability to fully appreciate its place and importance. Then again, in a culture devoid of depth and ingrained spirituality, maybe this is not a surprise. I know he also sees the use of medication here to be very limited, and maybe for emergency use only. But I also know he sees all such medication that affects the mind by modulating the brain to be a very blunt instrument; more like using a hammer and ice pick to fix the brain, I think he said.

Kennan is also of the belief that the complex of wounding, trauma, and stress is fundamental to understanding illness and disease from a true causal position. He sees a kind of cascade effect, where a psychic shock moves through the mind and then the body, explaining the resulting range of effects on both mind and body over time. The failure to recognise this leads to limited and often inappropriate management.

At this deeper level, we need counsel and guidance of a more psychospiritual nature. Otherwise, the danger is that the events are destined to repeat, or lead to a range of illnesses and diseases, inevitably and somewhat predictably. Maybe in the next chapter, where we will look at some specific health problems, this outline may become more apparent and practical.

Seventeen

It could be difficult to discuss specific medical conditions without lapsing into a list categorised by modern western medicine itself. I asked Kennan how he would approach such a task. He felt that maybe the best way was to start off with some general principles that took the emphasis more toward or even from a fundamentally holistic perspective, and then move through specific problems with these themes running through the exposition. He also believed that the focus should be on problems that were current and significant in the community, maybe not well dealt with, and more responsive to different viewpoints. Obviously, this list would not be exhaustive, but I understood from this that what might emerge would be a way any reader could look at and address problems not specifically covered here.

What I understand from all this is that one of the problems is translation. What we generally do is see a problem, illness or disease as defined by and in MWM's terms. Then we try to translate it, rather than looking at it afresh. We often do this when engaging complementary and alternative medicine, when we compare the new viewpoint with the one that MWM has already given us, instead of taking the new viewpoint on its own terms. These 'terms' often mean understanding the philosophy – often of a spiritual nature – in which other approaches are embedded. If this philosophy does not sit well with the patient, even after stripping away the western medical worldview, it is unlikely a differing approach will work anyway. Also, sometimes we try and translate, not just the problem, but also any different viewpoint back into MWM's terms. All in all, there are various levels and directions of translation required; the phrase "lost in the translation" readily comes to mind.

Kennan believes this process of change, or what he and others refer to as the paradigm shift that is engaging medicine, should be understood more fundamentally. We should get away from the prejudice of our conditioning and examine health issues with new eyes and on their own terms. Of course, this is difficult to do, particularly when fear enters the picture; but it may be essential for a creative change to be effective. He is also quite disparaging of medical terminology that distances health problems, sometimes deliberately from the patient, by objectifying them. And, of course, this is reinforced by the reliance on objective criteria – such as pathology, radiology and investigations in general – that create even further distance and objectification. Cancer becomes 'the' cancer, it is no longer 'my' cancer, the one 'I' have and must deal with.

We are in the early stage of this paradigm shift, believes Kennan, but he is certain that we are now actually in it. We know that with certain health problems, including the ones outlined in this chapter, we have yet to grasp a different way of looking at, embracing, and understanding them. But in spite of these difficulties, it is something we must begin and try to do. To the reader, this may appear as an incomplete process and that the problem cannot as yet be redefined, so there will be a tendency to lapse back on what we already know – or think that we know.

Kennan's response, as highlighted in this chapter, is that in many cases – maybe the majority – we do not properly understand many of the problems that we purport to, and that this brute realisation on his behalf is the subject matter of much of this account. But there are a lot of hints and alternative evidence that not only indicate that we may have the present picture as defined by MWM wrong, but we are on a path to finding other ways to envisage it; which, in turn, influences how we manage the many illnesses and diseases that are patently not responding to MWM's viewpoints and treatments.

I also realise now, and as a result of our exchanges, that there are some more general positions about health, which we must include from the onset. Kennan is adamant that the profession is actively resisting many of these positions, rather like the little Dutch boy sticking his fingers in the cracks of the dyke, even as the overwhelming tide beyond threatens further. I know he also believes that even though a holistic position is inclusive of the practitioner, the health setting, and the metaphysical aspects of medicine, it is probably better to engage MWM inclusively in the realm of health modelling, at present. He also believes this is a fundamental mistake made by many of a complementary, alternative, or new age persuasion; they are unable or unwilling to dialogue with and challenge MWM directly, often because the practitioners themselves have not made the full 'translation' described a little earlier.

Fundamental to this is that the medical model of health used by MWM is skewed toward pathology and does not include physiology sufficiently. Reversing this would mean that the practitioner would rely more on nature, the body with its healing and balancing mechanisms – known and unknown – than he or she presently does. But to do this demands patience, trust, and the ability to resist reacting to fear. It is in the nature of healing that an illness often gets worse – apparently – before it gets better – the so-called 'healing crisis'.

Kennan is also of the opinion that the knowledge employed by MWM is often restricted, distorted, or actively excludes other positions. There are many inherent faults in the reasoning behind such commonly used information, such as that derived from double-blind trials and statistical methods; maybe too many to account for here. Yet this is the basis of the so-called evidence-based medicine that is touted as fundamental in deriving medical knowledge. The perceptive reader will have noted the references to other agencies about this point, most particularly the pharmaceutical industry, and recognise many other concerning aspects of their involvement in the present picture of the way medical knowledge and thus ongoing education is derived.

We also need to recognise that knowledge changes over time; it always has. To believe that we are on the ultimate path to some fixed and permanent foundational knowledge, championed by science, is naïve and even dangerous. To only accept changes of knowledge that satisfy certain restricted definitions is small-minded and an intellectual insult. Yet MWM is guilty on both counts and more.

Kennan has frequently highlighted two significant domains we have yet to integrate into the current MWM model. The first he believes it is possible for medicine to integrate, and is beginning to do so, even though at present on its own terms only. The second he believes will be a more significant tool for the actual paradigm shift and medicine's redefinition.

The first is the role of nutrition, exercise, and mental attitude in health. These old archetypal stalwarts are making a return, and not before time. However, nutrition has not as yet recognised its involvement with the second domain, to which we will come soon, and restricting itself to a somewhat exclusively scientific approach. Exercise is being appreciated as well, even though it suffers from excessive scientific rigour. Attitude is similarly restricted to a psychological understanding with such phrases as 'positive thinking'. Attitude is much more than this; it opens to the realm of values and beliefs, as well as meaning and purpose. Ultimately, it is a spiritual concern and diminished by being looked at only cognitively and psychologically.

The second promised domain is the environment, specifically

environmental poisoning. This is where nutrition overlaps both domains, because it suffers from much poisoning beyond straightforward food manufacturing. Yet our homes – kitchens, bathrooms and laundries – are full of poisons, both in the structure of the house and the contents we bring into these areas. We apply poisons to our skin, body and mouth. We wash and shower in treated water, and we drink it. We are poisoned electromagnetically as well as industrially in our cars, offices, and workplaces. When our total climate is poisoned, how can we avoid it?

The effect these various poisons have on both body and mind is monstrous and immoral. I will mention – again – the pharmaceutical industry here, as well as such concerns about vaccination from the poisoning viewpoint alone. The role of additives, preservatives and in food, flavourings and colourings, are still not adequately recognised or evaluated properly.

So, with all these caveats in mind, maybe it is time to move on to some concrete examples. As we do this, I will be trying to weave in the points outlined immediately above, to illustrate not only their relevance, but that their inclusion is essential in the knowledge that will result within the paradigm change.

Type 2 diabetes ticks many of the above boxes. It is a good example of where a diagnosis is inappropriately used, when a syndrome better defines the phenomenon. It is also a modern phenomenon; a product of our pseudo-affluent western lifestyle. It is usually diagnosed by an investigation – and a very old and cumbersome one at that – the two-hour glucose tolerance test. Yet it confuses two phenomena: The first is the now rarer form, when the pancreas gland that produces the insulin that metabolises sugar in the body simply wears out. In this case, there is often a family history or genetic pattern in this and, in spite of all attempts to reverse it with diet and exercise, medication and insulin injections usually become necessary over time.

The second form of type 2 diabetes that has become an epidemic is associated with weight gain and high cholesterol levels, as fats are manufactured from sugar in the body, when the latter is not immediately utilised. Sugar levels then progressively rise over time, blood pressure may be raised, and the patient is often poor in the exercising department. What is less well known is that chronic stress can lead to raised sugar levels on a regular basis and ultimately on to diabetes. This picture is really a syndrome and some have called it Syndrome X, although Metabolic Syndrome is a better descriptor.

What can be seen from this very brief and condensed outline is that type 2 diabetes, better described as metabolic syndrome and currently in epidemic proportion, is a direct product of most, if not all, of the lifestyle factors described earlier in this chapter. It was uncommon when Kennan qualified. It starts as metabolic imbalance leading to physiological disturbance that, if chronic and persistent, produces potentially irreversible changes such as insulin resistance, where the insulin the pancreas gland produces fails to metabolise sugar and leads to raised blood sugar levels. It does not require a medical degree to understand this, nor to work out how to manage it.

As a brief aside, as recently as 300 years ago, sugar was seen as a drug. Maybe we should still see it that way. Our refining of complex carbohydrates to simple ones creates havoc with a system that is used to complex ones only, as well as leading to all sorts of fatigue and stress states, eating disorders and other medical problems, most notably heart disease. Kennan believes it is both directly and indirectly strongly associated with cancer.

In Kennan's view, sugar is more responsible for heart disease than cholesterol ever was or will be. The rise in cholesterol levels is a consequence of excess sugar in the diet initially, and subsequently the failure to metabolise it. Sugar and other environmental poisons, toxins, and the consequent inflammation are directly responsible for blood vessel disease; hence heart attacks, strokes, and vascular disease. Fats, specifically cholesterol, then build up on the blood vessel wall in an attempt to neutralise the toxicity (poisoning) and inflammation, and stop the vessels becoming further damaged. But it cannot do this indefinitely and, in the process, we wrongly identify cholesterol as the culprit. Kennan's earlier remarks about and description of chelation therapy should be read in this context.

As should Kennan's comments about trauma and wounding. Because we live under the chronic wounding that stress can produce. Not only is diabetes a result but also, and for similar reasons, so is heart disease of the degenerative variety. This then brings in the mental health side of the picture and, from a holistic perspective, factors like occupational history and the role of the environment. Stress also compounds inflammation in a number of ways, direct and indirect. Blood pressure, an independent risk factor for heart disease and not a disease itself, is also raised by stress. So, it should be no surprise that the reduction of blood pressure with medication alone is misleading; firstly, blood pressure is not primarily a disease and, secondly, medication may reduce the blood pressure but not the issues – like stress – that produce it in the first place, so masking these deeper issues.

In simple terms, it is all a question of 'too little, too late', plus the inability or lack of resolve to deal with the extensive, deep, and significant background that is either ignored or not adequately addressed. These are modern diseases, as I have noted here and elsewhere, and modern medicine is both a product of the factors that have led to them, as well as being inadequate in their management. This is a vast area and our knowledge is incomplete, although there is definitely more available than the medical profession acknowledges. Yet, if you track the argument above, it can be seen that management and, more particularly prevention, is not rocket science and is freely available.

Using pharmaceutical drugs in this domain is fraught with problems. Using a drug when non-drug approaches – like diet and exercise – are more fundamentally effective and with fewer side effects, is simply bad medicine. In the case of blood pressure medication, it can mask the reasons that blood pressure is raised in the first place, and in the case of cholesterol-lowering medications, it is based on inadequate knowledge and little applied wisdom. It should not be forgotten that cholesterol is largely manufactured in the body and is also essential for hormone production including, ironically, the stress hormone that is produced in response to stressors.

Although type 2 diabetes is technically a hormonal disease, because insulin is a hormone, it is really a metabolic problem and should be primarily treated metabolically. Ideally, it should be prevented by lifestyle issues in the first place, so avoiding its onset. It is always easier and better for one's health to prevent rather than to manage a problem.

Other hormonal problems can overlap this very broad picture, as can be seen with stress, cholesterol, and the health of the adrenal glands that manage stress in the body. The attentive reader may recall that Kennan had a diagnosis of diabetes and much that I have written above applies to his changed understanding of it as a primary disease and most certainly its management. It should never be forgotten that alteration of hormonal environments in a haphazard manner has all sorts of consequences for mental and sexual health.

The way we describe the body indicates how we look at it and its contents, even governing our perspective. In general, medicine views the body reductively, separating out organs and glands. From there, it describes how each component looks (anatomy) and works (physiology). So, we have the heart or brain described as organs, and the pancreas or adrenals as glands (a gland secretes something). Yet we also recognise that these organs and glands can be part of an interconnected system, such as the cardiovascular or nervous systems, or described more by its function, such as the metabolic or stress-response systems.

When we describe systems, we are starting to look more holistically. The nervous system is conceptually broader and larger than the brain. Sometimes this picture becomes more nebulous, such as with the stress response and its extension to the immune system, which is quite difficult to conceive of in our structured and mechanical worldview. Also, these more complex systems respond less well to medical intervention, which should come as no surprise; they are more fluid and connected with emotions and mental states, as well as a broader and more holistic view.

In Kennan's opinion, it is systems like the immune and hormonal ones that most demonstrate the limitations of the current MWM worldview. Trying to extend this worldview into territory that can't be defined in this way is intellectual sloppiness; we should be trying to reconceive how we view them, particularly when the current management for illness and disease in these systems is so woefully inadequate and sometimes counterproductive to the overall welfare of the body.

Kennan's view is much more fluid and process-oriented. He is always concerned to see how and when dysfunction occurs and then follow its pathway into illness and disease. He believes we will then better understand the diseases that we are currently dealing with inadequately, and maybe ultimately all disease, in this manner. He refers to it as a top-down approach, with beginnings in the metaphysical realms, including the mind and emotions, as well as soul and spirit. Then the progression is through specific systems, most notably the nervous system ('mind'), but not excluding the cardiovascular system ('heart'). From there the radiation is into the various bodily systems and to the organs within them. Not surprisingly, this contains his aforementioned views on shock, stress, trauma and wounding.

This perspective gives a more inclusive way of looking at some modern problems, such as autoimmune disease. For example, Kennan frequently refers to autoimmune thyroiditis, commonly called Hashimoto's disease after its identifier, that commonly leads to a poorly functioning thyroid gland, known as hypothyroidism. He points out that this form of thyroiditis is highly inflammatory and primarily an immune system problem, prior to considering it as a hormone or glandular one. It is also different from the type of hypothyroidism where the gland itself simply ceases to function; he sees parallels with type 2 diabetes here and even discerns a general principle.

In this case, it is easy to distinguish the two types of hypothyroidism, as in the clinical picture the gland of thyroiditis is swollen and tender because of inflammation, and a blood test can determine that the immune system is acting inappropriately toward the thyroid gland. It is as if the immune system is attacking the thyroid, as it would a foreign organ like a transplant, but here it is acting against itself.

Kennan, unsurprisingly, sees this as a metaphor of a deeper problem and traces it back to stress and the nervous system … and beyond. He then sees how this both influences and reorientates treatment. The common way is to treat the end result, the poorly functioning thyroid, with a replacement hormone called thyroxine. Not only is this synthetic, it is probably not the hormone to use. Rather, a naturally derived hormone mixture that is the same as the thyroid's normal output should be used in a supplemental manner; that is, not controlling or replacing the normal output but merely supporting it, otherwise the thyroid will not recover over time and stop working completely.

Not only does Kennan consider this a shame, it is unnecessary. The main focus should be to support the immune system and the resultant inflammation that focuses on the thyroid gland. This also requires – as do so many of the diseases in this autoimmune category – attention to healthy bowel functioning; a lot, if not all, inflammatory diseases can be traced back to this source or at least involve it in management.

There is also an argument that all such autoimmune system disorders, called diseases, can be traced back to a preceding tendency, pattern of behaviour, problem or trauma should we adopt a more metaphoric and even symbolic view of illness and disease. Kennan believes this area represents a lot of exciting challenges and is keen for patients to be able to actively learn how to look at their problems this way. He sees this as the healing pathway that supervenes and includes any mechanical attempt to deal with and fix the problem.

It is also concerning how many diseases are now being identified as autoimmune, and the number is increasing. Of most notable interest to Kennan are the nervous system ones, like multiple sclerosis. He also believes this represents the challenging end of the spectrum to MWM and where the points of intersection with a holistic medical worldview may have a creative outcome to the progress and future of the paradigm shift.

In all this, though, we have to be careful not to become too introverted. Although, given that we live in an extraverted world and blame all things 'outside' and 'elsewhere' for our problems, this is not in itself a bad thing. But we do need to balance the emotion, mind, and soul perspective with the deeper external influences of our diet, the environment, our occupations, and loss of family and social cohesion.

It is not surprising that Kennan views cancer as a simple extension of the above discussion and arguments. Recall that he has a personal and very intimate connection with cancer, and is one of few people in his position to also see its progress without the normal interventions that MWM confers. It has given him extraordinary insights into cancer as a phenomenon, but he is very wary about the company with which he shares these for what, by now, should be some obvious reasons.

All the points to date are equally applicable to cancer, even though they may appear more urgent to those afflicted and immediately involved, such as family and friends. He is quite adamant that history will judge the use of surgery, radiotherapy, and chemotherapy very poorly, and to be quite misguided. He is also quite aware of the vested interests, at many levels, that fail to tackle the problem in what he sees as some obvious ways. He does not deny the input of genetic and other research, but believes it is still just that – research – and we have to be careful how and when we apply it as treatment.

Kennan is also intrigued by the personality and psychological patterns that stand behind cancer; indeed, immune diseases in general. He also distinguishes genetic insights that are physical from those that may represent deep psychological patterns; because, if nothing else, the latter demand a quite different approach. But he is fascinated by some commentators who see cancer as some primitive attempt at healing, and that this is a line of inquiry that reflects and parallels his more metaphysical understandings and their input. In my eyes, this is the stuff of workshops, and I am not surprised that he became quite circumspect about detail and speculation here beyond a certain point.

Kennan's own position is that there is no single cause to cancer; there may be triggers, but to see a simple cause and effect pattern is simplistic and does not fit the evidence. Instead, cancer needs revisioning: He sees that there is chain of events from the subtle to the manifest by the time a mass is detected in an organ or gland. Cancer is multifactorial in its genesis and only a truly holistic approach will encompass these varying factors. He feels that such ignored disciplines as embryology may have some bearing on the manifestation process, and that these point to the earlier comment that cancer may be some sort of healing process that we misinterpret and therefore mistreat.

This position makes Kennan very wary of interpreting the findings of so-called early detection procedures. In addition to his earlier concerns, he believes they often do more harm than good and may ultimately be found to have little bearing on outcome; instead, creating much in the way of physical and mental morbidity. We have also closed the door to seeing the life history of cancer and its outcome; our predictions therefore become detrimental to all concerned, and often a death sentence – akin to 'pointing the bone' – to the patient.

Kennan has given examples of his thinking within our discussions and we have gone down many a track in this exploration. He has paid particular attention to cancers of the brain, sex glands and organs, as well as specific cancers like melanoma in this process. We discussed the value of translating these discussions to this account, but both felt this is not appropriate. To lay out controversial viewpoints in a more specific manner could be detrimental to a potential sufferer reading this account, without the necessary back up and support. He is adamant that such dialogue and discussion be confined to appropriate settings.

It intrigues me that Kennan has come to the position that he has with medicine generally, and physical health specifically, after a long sojourn in mental health and depth psychology. Even during this sojourn, it seems he never lost contact with the body, as he believed many psychiatrists had done. Although there is some redress going on in the profession presently, it is a long way from achieving some sort of mind-body reunification. In Kennan's opinion, this unity is a given and medicine may struggle to progress without it. In his mind, its reintegration may even be the indicator that the new paradigm is upon us.

Kennan sees his views to embrace both physical medicine and mental health. While he knows there is no such specific thing as a mental disease, he believes we must reconceive both the mind in health and even so-called diseases of the brain. Intuitively, he believes that we are a long way from understanding diseases like Parkinson's, and that they represent a window into worlds we need to explore, prior to or as well as the mechanical and potentially mind-numbing pharmacological approaches that we routinely take.

In a wider sense, Kennan sees that mental health should actually not be the province of medicine as it stands, nor psychiatry specifically. He is of the opinion that we are in danger of losing sight of the thrust and approaches that depth psychology undertook in the last century, but understands that the risks taken in these fields would not be tolerated presently. Yet he sees this as a shame and stifling of exploration. Leaving mental health in the hands of psychiatry and the pharmaceutical industry may even threaten us as a species, he believes.

Kennan sees a more expansive position for mental distress, in a view of mental health that connects us with all levels of our existence as human beings. We are as yet a long way from such a unified position, as professionally we are a race of specialists. There must be more blending between scientific disciplines and the relativity of science itself appreciated; medicine must also see itself in this wider context. There should be more discussion and dialogue with less argument and conflict. We need to integrate the more fundamental instinctual and emotional aspects of ourselves into a more holistic perspective, so that our prejudices and preconceptions do not govern our progress as a species. We need to understand ourselves as spiritual beings.

There could be more I could discuss about mental health and illness, as well as Kennan's view of these; but as they make up a continuing theme of this work, I may be in danger of repeating him, and also myself. Instead, it may be of value to see the application of these views in various other areas of medicine.

Kennan understands that, as a species, we are somewhere within the predator-prey spectrum. In fact, we are under an illusion that we are somehow the top dog and no longer susceptible to being the prey, as would be apparent in our evolutionary history. This illusion may also lead to our imagining prey, such as alien abductors, or may distort the view we take of the most common interaction we have at this level, with infectious disease.

Because of the lack of obvious predators, and our illusory isolation of ourselves within our own skin, we tend to view all other autonomous agents – viruses, bacteria, fungi, worms – as threats to our wellbeing and even our existence. That this can induce stress – a disordered immune response and inflammation as a consequence – should not be ignored. But are these autonomous agents really such a threat? Or, because we can't generally see them, are they like aliens or even threatening in the way an abnormal blood test is?

There is no doubt that these agents have been the scourge of history, with diseases like the plague decimating whole populations. A brief examination of early medical history, Greek, Roman, and even Anglo-Saxon, shows the attention paid to infectious agents. Yet one of the major turnarounds in the twentieth century was the reduction of threat with good nutrition, housing, and sanitation … well before the advent of antibiotics, I should remind the reader.

To gain a more balanced picture Kennan commonly outlines what 'bugs' do for our benefit. He cites the many kilos of them that inhabit the bowel and provide a dynamic environment for our healthy digestion and ultimate well-being. We most notice this when this environment is decimated by antibiotics. He also points to the role of fungi in the discovery of penicillin, to balance the negative perception of their overgrowth when bacteria are killed by antibiotics; pointing out that the fungi are growing simply to fill a void left after the antibiotic insult. There is something circular and more than a little ironic when fungi are seen this way.

Kennan also believes that routine childhood illnesses, like chicken pox, may provide levels of immunity in adult life to other problems. He wonders how much this neglect is a factor in auto-immune disease and even cancer. He also, unsurprisingly, questions the manner and degree with which we employ vaccination to appease our fears, rather than for our fundamental wellbeing. To illustrate this, he points out that the original vaccination – using cowpox to prevent smallpox – is really an extension of agricultural life amongst the animals, as well as the role of lesser childhood infections in immunity.

Whilst the arguments in these areas are complex and varied, the actual principles are quite simple and easy to grasp. We just have to overcome some psychological hurdles, such as pre-conception and prejudice, to listen to them. And this does not stop with infectious agents; consider bee stings and even snake bites as agents of immunity. As humans, and like stress, it seems we thrive and grow from these challenges. It is in our nature.

We also need to understand infectious diseases more fundamentally prior to our reliance on vaccination or pharmaceutical agents. Rather like climate change, but perhaps greater than it, Kennan sees the use of agents like antibiotics in the blatantly misguided and inappropriate manner in which they are currently used to be a threat to at least the future generations, if not ourselves. It seems to him, because we have lost our more fundamental position and role on the planet, we may be in danger of self-extinction prior to the imagined threatened one to us from outside.

To extend on the pharmaceutical argument, and avoiding the other nefarious concerns about the industry itself, is also a principle that cuts across the spectrum. Kennan nominates drugs in the treatment of mental health and pain as being the most notable and concerning in – ironically – causing more mental illness and suffering from pain. We are a long way, it seems, from grasping the full significance of what we are doing with pharmacy. In his terminology, the gods, through mystical alchemy, have given us a powerful tool and we are misusing it to our potential destruction. Strong words indeed.

The examination of the role of pharmacy extends into another contentious area: Iatrogenic, or medically-caused disease, which may be the third highest cause of death in the western world. Iatrogenic disease is usually related to treatment, although it can also be due to examination processes, such as an adverse radiological event. Of the many thousands of deaths due to iatrogenesis every year, conservatively estimated to be over 10,000 in Australia, the majority are drug errors of various kinds. Second in line are hospital infections, where drugs also have an obvious part to play. Third is unnecessary surgery and hospital errors generally. Across the spectrum, hospital treatments predominate – not healthy places to visit, it seems.

We have covered the patterns in drugs, infections, and hospitals at various points in this account, but when they are put together in this combined manner, then maybe more than anything else, iatrogenesis points to all not being well with MWM. Iatrogenesis could even be seen as a metaphor for the current medical paradigm being terminal.

I want to add a postscript about the medical encounter between doctor and patient that Kennan and I have decided to include more as an afterthought. Initially, Kennan felt that it should really be part of his educational delivery, but as we have progressed through this account, he told me that – even if only in a summary form – he would like it included here, too.

Classically, when a doctor first encounters a patient, he or she takes a medical history. That is the complaint is asked for, a history of its development elucidated, and then any past relevant medical history asked for. If any drugs or medications are used, this is entered, then the family and social histories are asked. These latter two are often given scant attention and generally ignored in a brief encounter, or registered in other ways, by a nurse assistant, for example.

Kennan's inclination would now be to reverse this process and to see the narrative around the disorder to emerge from the social, environmental, occupational and family histories. This reversal reminds me of the way that Kennan sees the physical to be embedded in greater and progressively more subtle realities, as in the perennial philosophy or great chain of being.

But more than this, Kennan inclines to the patient developing their own narrative, with appropriate questions surely, as a life story in which the problem is embedded and arises over time. Not only does this capture elements otherwise excluded and hence be more holistic and less reductive, it also gives authority back to the patient, if conducted well. As he sees such factors as patient self-responsibility, empowerment and control to be essentials in the healing process, it is well to encourage them from the very beginning.

However, there is a wider dimension to this; that is, connecting the patient to his or her own symptoms more fundamentally. In this way, the patient is 'listening' to their own story and may come to an understanding of its origins, nature and even treatment. The present problem may then serve as a template for future ones.

The words over a century ago of William Osler, the Canadian physician, ring true here: "Listen to your patient; he is telling you the diagnosis." In psychotherapy, there is a shift of emphasis from the shamanic appreciation of soul retrieval undertaken by the medicine man, to one where the client undertakes this under the guidance and mentorship of the shaman. I believe this is a general principle and would modify the quote to: "If you let your patient talk long enough, and you listen properly, they will tell you what's wrong with them", and maybe not need your services anyway!

Eighteen

I had thought that maybe this was a good place to stop. I had even moved into the present in the more recent writing, so as to bring the account relatively up to date and thus anticipate some sort of closure. However, external circumstances beyond our immediate sphere of concern were to supersede that demanded our attention.

We both stepped back from our meetings around this work to let it settle, prior to finalisation. However, events across the board – family, business and professional – were to emerge for Kennan in rapid succession. I then had a recent, though not unsurprising cancer diagnosis to negotiate. Then, in early 2020 Covid emerged and our completion was pushed back even further. Kennan felt that all these events would need some sort of inclusion and integration to bring the work to a conclusion.

A further reason for this has been that spiritually Kennan has become deeply drawn into the story of Merlin and the subsequent myths and legends around the Arthurian narrative, most specifically the Holy Grail. He began writing about this recently after researching and exploring this territory over a long period, ever since he discovered Jung, in fact. He then realised that the last three or so years to the present needed accounting for in this work before he could comfortably proceed with the proposed *Charm of Making* that was about Merlin and the Grail legends.

In effect, this planned work of the *Charm of Making* was to be his third and final with a strong memoir and legacy component. He had written and privately published the cheekily titled, *The*

Porn User's Guide to Enlightenment, in the realms of what he calls psychosexuality and its relationship to spirituality; the present work with its focus on medicine being the second. All three works aimed to ground major areas of life experience into a personal perspective, so making them more relatable and understanding to people who did not know him, to provide more insight and access for their own personal development. Being part-educational in nature, part personally therapeutic, and by increasing awareness of and in these fields, he hoped to contribute to opening up areas that had been and continue to be difficult to access.

In this process, I have decided to insert the events of these three or so years here in this account. But I have left the last chapter of a concluding perspective, written by Kennan prior to Covid, relatively untouched. This is because it provides a personal end statement of closure that still manages to encompass these subsequent three or so years, but also because it is perennial, prophetic, and even archetypal, touching on what he sees as the bedrock of medicine. The written account from this point to the beginning of the concluding chapter resulted from our resumed and ultimately final meetings.

I began the discussion with Kennan:

"I recall that your father's death in 2018 had an indirect but rather reverberating effect on you; it wasn't long after that we kind of suspended our meetings around this account, thinking it was relatively complete. However, as I recall, I had left it up to you to initiate the finalisation process?" This was a summarising statement, as much for any audience as Kennan, who rarely required such a detailed provocation.

"Quite right," was the immediate response. "I don't feel that Phil's death had a big impact on me, although I am possibly not the best person to judge. More significant was that, during this same period, shortly after his death, my colleague and writing collaborator on the Traditional Medicine Ways course, Rafael, also passed away. Although Rafael and I had drifted somewhat for several years, there had been a strong psychic and brotherly bond, even love between us. In these later years, I had taken this collaboration elsewhere with you in this work, then you were diagnosed about the time of Rafael's death, which is also when my marriage had really begun to flounder.

"I started to feel quite alone and isolated, although a lot of this was self-imposed. I did not have the heart to work on and complete this account, as you knew from our own relationship beyond these specific meetings. Instead, I felt I must attend to my marriage. Added to this, the business I had invested in to fund the home retreat's development also started to have financial difficulties. My reading of this was that the opportunity it had demonstrated had passed by, and it was now terminal. Things were generally not looking good, but I felt I had to put my energy into all of these factors and see how to progress."

Although, of course, I knew all this, the sheer magnitude of it when laid out so succinctly and raw still struck me. I was also aware that he was attending to his core practice of psychotherapy to put food on the table, and not extending much into the prior educational and teaching domains, even with my prompting. As Rafael had been his main support and collaborator in this area, it was not surprising. But at a deeper level, I wondered whether these intersecting forces would finally overwhelm him and detract from his intention and commitment to further the development of medicine in the modern era more broadly. I also asked myself, why is this happening? Hadn't there been enough challenges to afford him peace and reflection, or were there further demands being made of him? Or, somewhat more pessimistically, was he somehow missing the point about his life, direction and purpose?

I also felt that there were two themes operating from this time that I could draw on. The first was Kennan's own health challenges, being generally the lifelong infectious illness, ones up to and including the viral pneumonia of 2016. With the advent of Covid, we could both now clearly identify this as severe acute respiratory syndrome, or SARS; a kind of Covid precursor that makes Kennan's appreciation of the latter more intimate. He was also to have a specific health challenge during this three-year period, just as Covid started, which was to have more of a dramatic impact on him. There were also the past traumas and the associated stresses to consider. Not only had Kennan's direct experience linked the two, but James had even diagnosed it as PTSD. Kennan, however, was disinclined to use the latter acronym, as he felt it facilitated too much in the way of victim psychology rather than seeing the contributing events as part of his life journey.

The second theme was a bit more problematic from my perspective, as it indicated this three-year period contained three phases; death, the underworld journey (or dark night of the soul), and resurrection. In other words, there was an archetypal theme operating. Maybe, I thought, this is why some of the questions I posed had not been answered; at least, until this point. Maybe Kennan had not fully identified the core of himself, his heart or soul, and required these more extreme measures to realise this. In this way, they could be considered part of his fate, his wyrd, and that it was almost inevitable he would bring them upon himself.

Covid will weave itself through both themes and even unite them in a holistic manner, or so it seemed to me. So, here in its barest chronological outline is the skeleton of events that occurred in this three-year period that includes both themes, but uses the second – death, underworld, resurrection – to begin to flesh out this skeleton, before we move into the specifics of the medical problems that comprise the first.

After the events of 2018, themselves pointing to death, Kennan recalls a clear evening at dinner early in 2019 where and when he realised that his wife no longer wanted the marriage to continue and neither now did he. This was because with the children now grown, she wanted to stay in the city with her extended family, whereas he wanted to return to the south and the fledgling retreat. Although the retreat was still in their possession at that time, Kennan felt compromised; he knew that the process he was to unleash meant that the property may be reclaimed by the bank anyway, but he knew his wife wanted nothing to do with it. With all this, he realised his marriage was ending.

Over the coming year, the business supporting the property failed and, with default of repayments, the bank reclaimed the property. Also, and by mutual agreement, the marriage formally ended toward the end of the year. At this time, Kennan actually experienced his heart 'breaking' in a physical manner and, for the next few months, he knew he was playing Russian roulette with a heart that was now out of rhythm; but he seemed not to care. This built to a head when one day in early 2020 he saw that he could either die or actively intervene and continue to live. It felt like a close call, but he put himself in the hands of his profession and used medication to correct the rhythm, but declined the recommended ongoing and permanent medicalisation that went with it.

Covid was just hitting the city, so he decided to leave. Lighter of baggage, he went to live for over a year in a small den on a property next to an old-growth forest region of the State's southwest. Death now became underworld. He settled into a rhythm of long walks, good diet and supplementation, no alcohol or medication and lots – and lots – of reflection and contemplation. Nature was his healer, his nurturing; he reconnected in a fundamental manner with these patterns of his childhood but with a conviction about 'country' and this new land as home. Days were spent without talking to anyone. He maintained a skeleton of his counselling and therapy practice, now online with the occasional local seeking him out, but relied on a pension as the bank sought a purchaser for the former home retreat.

It was a personally confronting time, sometimes quite brutal. He fast-tracked the grief of the loss of both marriage and property, although somewhat strangely, the latter did not engage much of the anticipated emotional pain, and this left him a bit quizzical. Yet he put this to one side as he proceeded through divorce, settlement, and selection of who in his life would comprise his future in any sort of social and professional sense.

By comparison, Covid and its effects seemed almost peripheral; in a strange sense he was unaffected, now seeing that his SARS illness of 2016 was almost a presentiment: SARS is, after all, a corona virus infection. But it gave him prior experience of the illness that was now epidemic, such that he felt he stood apart from it and saw, not only the medical but also the political, social and economic management and its distortions: It did not look good to him, driven as it was by dishonesty, duplicity and vested interests. Yet he had no desire to enter the fray, nor did he want to position himself in either of the two opposing and sometimes warring camps that had – predictably – evolved. Quite a powerful virus, he reflected.

Covid begins to wane and society itself begins to recover; but has it transformed? The early signs are not good. But what of Kennan, does he feel different? All the external markers indicate this, but I wondered how he felt in his heart, within his soul.

"There are several facets to the viral pneumonia – SARS – illness I had. Certainly, the way Covid is described with any respiratory involvement is very similar; in fact, the same. Interestingly, my wife and a couple of others in our Bali party had the temperatures, sore throat and the like, but I was the only one who then developed a lung problem. It was nasty; hurt like hell whenever I breathed – which was pretty frequently of course – and I felt clogged up, which made for anxiety as well." Kennan's account was fairly straightforward but made interesting because of the advent of Covid.

"It was the tiredness that really got me, the lack of any will. This was something I hadn't experienced before. I was ill with the amoebic parasite illness, but not so tired as this. It was almost as if I had no desire to live. So, when Covid came along I simply ran for cover. I did not want to risk exposure in the early days and I also didn't want to have what I consider to be experimental vaccination. An additional factor was that my heart event, which had occurred in the weeks preceding the pandemic outbreak, had a potential thrombosis component and my early understanding of Covid and the vaccination was that this was an unnecessary risk.

"The heart event was pivotal in a psychological and spiritual way, but fairly straightforward from the physical perspective. The experience I had of a broken heart was of the physical sensation of my heart region being physically split open … I didn't think that it was pain, as in a heart attack. Then there was an upwelling of intense emotion that was almost indescribable in terms of what it specifically felt like; it was core, primal. The whole episode lasted about twenty minutes, I guess, and occurred on a walk I had in a park neighbouring where my wife and I lived: I was actually on my way to our last meeting, where and when we decided to separate. Although I knew it was the right thing to do, I was still absolutely gutted.

"From that point my heart rhythm became odd. There were periods it was okay, but then it would be very fast and sometimes quite irregular. I knew what was going on, but I was grieving intensely and being pursued by the bank and others from the now failed business, as I had been a loan guarantor amongst my other involvements. All these issues conflated and, as anyone knows who has been through something similar, the various agencies do not leave you alone. I was again playing Russian roulette, it seemed, but I didn't seem to care.

"Then after a few months, I developed chest pain. I suspected it was my deceased father Phil's home-made wine plus poor eating, but I saw it as an opportunity to either "stay or go". I was living at my parents' now vacated house in the city, as my mother had gone into care. In a matter of symbolic acting out, I had even placed a rope at the back door as a mind game. It did remind me of the suicides when I was a psychiatric registrar, however. I rolled the dice, called an ambulance and ended up in hospital, where my questionable heart attack was treated by getting my heart rhythm straight, prescribing a bunch of predictable medications, and then shown the door.

"I didn't have a heart attack. I knew that even at the time. The evidence was scant, based on a blood test result that might have been abnormal for other reasons such as the odd rhythm. The older nurses knew this, as I was being medically processed by the cardiologist. Instead, I respectively declined his proposed ongoing management and set about getting myself righted with the support and guidance of a GP friend, who was well aware of all these intersecting factors. I was also to discover that there was such a thing as Broken Heart Syndrome (BHS) and that I fitted the bill. Case closed. Covid arrives. I head to the den in the forest. The BHS was something I also realised I had not known about, nor did the cardiologist or other doctors I encountered.

"Whilst from a medical perspective this has now been well and truly negotiated and I am in a different physical place – fitter, leaner, wiser – it had an enormous psychic effect on me, with what was obviously a death wish standing behind the fear of dying. Coming out of hospital I found I had momentum and proceeded to actively deal with the loose ends of business, banks and finance. I decided to effectively clear my patch and shed all such attachments, realising that financially I was now on my own and could survive on relatively little. I also could see all the encumbrances we generally carry around with us and, although now far from completely shed, I went to the den a lot lighter, materially as well as psychically."

And that is how it sounds, I thought when I heard all this. There was something in Kennan's tone of voice, his expression and demeanour. Although I did have one question, and that was about alcohol usage. It has a theme that found its way, overtly and covertly, through the whole narrative.

"Interesting though not surprising you should ask about alcohol at this point, but I don't intend to go back through the places where it arises in my personal and also professional account to date. Now I would like to look at it a bit more deeply as the first theme you outlined at the beginning of this chapter, and include alcohol in that process.

"But first, some more about alcohol. Prior to their marriage, my mother, Ena, became accidentally pregnant to my father, which, of course, was socially a real no-no at this time just after the end of the Second World War. During the second trimester and late for this to be undertaken, as well as being illegal, my parents procured the services of a deregistered doctor who – apparently under the influence – initiated labour in a forest and left Ena in labour to deliver a dead child. This took three days to occur and the deceased male child, named Stephen, was duly buried in a field on her mother and father's farm.

"Given the circumstances at the time, none of this is

surprising, although the resonance with the doctor, his alcohol predilection and deregistered status, has a strange reverberation. I was the replacement for Stephen, although I was obviously reluctant, as it took Phil and Ena over a year to conceive me; it is interesting in that Stephen had presented no such difficulty. I found this out from Ena when I suspected – beyond the usual adoption fantasy common to many children – that something dark had occurred. Ena was surprisingly forthcoming, maybe it helped her conscience as Phil was not likely to have raised the matter again after it happened, which I later confirmed with him.

"Ena drank beer reasonably regularly, as I gather, during her pregnancy with me. I was born with the aid of forceps after a 36-hour labour, which Ena does not remember, as she had been given morphine. The GP doctor was known to be alcoholic. Phil was in the pub when the call came through to him. It was winter in England, mid-evening and very cold. Ena's first description of me was of seeing me in a crib and that I had a misshapen head (presumably due to the forceps), large hands and a birthmark on one knee. What struck me when Ena recounted this was the separation between she and I, and the problem-ridden description.

"In therapy as an adult, it was this description that alerted me to prior issues, such as Stephen, as well as the feeling that I was a replacement of sorts because I did not fit the bill. Stephen was described as beautiful and angelic … but dead. Not surprisingly, breastfeeding was a failure ("you were so angry") and we never really bonded, until maybe in adult life when we found a friendship, acceptance and ultimately love of each other. My younger sister – conceived seven months later after a boozy night out and apparently with no problem – had little in the way of intimate parenting, Ena having to wrestle with Phil's long-term marital indiscretion. Also, my sister lost half her hand in a farming accident when she was five.

"When I was just fifteen, Phil and his father, my grandfather, took me to the pub as some sort of initiation. I was filled with ale and spent half the night vomiting with a resulting hangover as a psychic trophy to take back to boarding school the next day. In spite of the hangover, the odd thing was I had a strange sense of feeling normal; had I some sort of 'Foetal Alcohol Syndrome'? Irrespective, the dye was cast and as a rugby player, well reinforced. Alcohol was an integral part of my social life. The rest you know, Ian, it is littered throughout this account in a narrative manner."

Although surprised by a lot of this account, I was not shocked. Somehow it all fitted into place. We discussed this a little further, but Kennan was keen to put the alcohol story into the theme structure we had formulated at the beginning of this chapter, prior to relating these further alcohol-related stories. A further round of coffee ensued.

"You will recall the other more archetypal theme of death, underworld and resurrection, of course. In effect, this is a "night sea journey" or a "dark night of the soul", if we listen to the accounts of some mystics. I liken it to a soul loss and retrieval process, somewhat shamanically. But this theme begs the question: Why is it even there in the first place and what sort of events bring about its necessity? However, and from the beginning I think it is important to realise that theme of the triggers for this process, which were outlined earlier in this chapter, are not commonly engaged as an initiatory path of transformation and 'soul retrieval' as described here. For most people, they become absolute events in and of themselves, and invested with all sorts of psychological accretions and outcomes that do not render them transformative.

"My classification that follows is based on the fact that we all face pain, suffering and trauma at some point or points in our life. So, this outline is to elaborate on what these are and in what context to put them, then the individual can refer them to the death-dark night of the soul-resurrection process I have outlined, and will continue to refer to.

"There are outer events, such as accidents or trauma, physical or psychological, though with inner ramifications. There are inner events, such as addictions, madness, and various disease processes. Then there are ones that are a bit of both, maybe infectious disease (external agent, internal immune state), cancer and various other illnesses, such as 'diseases of civilisation' (diabetes, heart disease). But it is important to remember that whilst we blame outer circumstances or feel guilty about inner ones, they all tend to flow in and out of each other in a dynamic fashion, rather like the eternity symbol or along a mobius strip, and also like the Yin-Yang symbol of eastern philosophy and mysticism.

"My own such challenges are littered throughout this narrative. Why we should seemingly have such challenges to face is more the province of mysticism, but it might be seen that it is tied up with transformation and, I believe, a kind of soul-making. I suspect there is something deeper at work here, being our relationship to the world of Spirit, as well as Spirit's desire and expectation of us. But the death experiences of a couple of years ago somehow felt to be the culmination of what preceded it, and maybe the reason we were unable to complete this account at that time, Ian."

I nodded in agreement, mainly as a feeling, because I was unsure about how much I was accurately following Kennan at this point. Or was it that he was also referring to what I was now going through?

"The next phase in the process was my fifteen months in the forest den. During this period, I spent a lot of my time and energy looking at what I had been through in the prior year or two, with considerable self-reflection and facing my own demons. I was also alcohol-free, although on a few occasions, I took some psilocybin in the form of naturally occurring mushrooms, finding the experiences very beneficial in the integration process and the ensuing stability of my psychological health. This is all a topic in its own right, but I mention it for the sake of completion, and also because I am an advocate of the use of such agents for mental distress.

"I also experienced some episodes of sleep paralysis that surprised and, at the time, frightened me. During these, I actually experienced my own birth and immediate perinatal circumstances. Whilst I had known these experiences before, it was only in an intellectual and mental manner. During this time, I went through the actual bodily experiences.

"I have resumed alcohol, initially socially with friends and intimate company, but have come to the conclusion it no longer serves the same purpose for me. In the latter stages prior to this period, I found I would drink heavily over a day or two to arrive at an altered state of consciousness, and then experience dreams and other psychic events. But the toll on my being was too harsh, particularly after the mushrooms. Alcohol also has many inherent dangers, some known physical ones, but also some less obvious spiritual ones. So, it is better now that I keep it to social occasions and ritual purposes, particularly as I have spontaneous access to the states I previously used it for.

"Am I resurrected? That is a bit presumptuous, but I am in a very different space from three to four years ago, and one I wouldn't have predicted. Much of my immediate past has fallen away, country engrosses me and I have aspects of my work and writing that continue, although in a less goal-directed and ambitious manner. But I do feel a distinct change and one that is more complete in a way that is different from any prior transitions.

"There is a sense of death containing no fear now, though

the challenge in front of me is to plumb its depths and significance for me. I also believe that I am operating much more naturally from a level I would term as soul, and can identify the self-in-the-world more distinctly, separately and readily. Also, I believe that this soul perspective has been discovered or uncovered through the various traumas I have been through, almost as if the process has made conscious what was only latently there previously and maybe could not have been revealed in any other way. My emotional and feeling states take precedence over my thinking and more mental processes now; I guess I now function more from my heart."

A quite gentle summary from Kennan, I thought, and a rather large statement to complete it. Given that the Covid pandemic had now generally passed in our State, I thought it was appropriate to get Kennan's views on this, as it had kind of paralleled and even mapped the last few years for him. I felt with his background that his insights would be useful and maybe helpful to many, although we were both keen to stay clear of any professional party line, conventional takes and socio-political interpretations.

Nineteen

Covid, apart from its nomination as an infectious pandemic, comprises one of the themes of pain and suffering Kennan has described; and it is both external and internal, affecting both physical and mental health. He considers the spectre of death is what has most driven it, so it simultaneously fits into the first phase of his archetypal triad of transformation, or soul retrieval. It is in this context that Kennan explores the Covid phenomenon and it is these insights that he wants to share, rather than the more medical, political or socially-driven ones. But what does Kennan mean here by the "the spectre of death"?

"In modernity, and in the absence of any meaningful religious structure and instead superseded by materialism, technology and the general false god of scientism, there is what I refer to as a 'hyper-individualised' sense of an existence defined by and confined to life experience between birth and death. We have lost our psychic bearings around issues like ancestry, lineage and tradition, which is reinforced by losing our necessary relationship to our creativity and spirituality. The instincts tend to rule from below an apparently encultured existence that is really wafer-thin; scratch it, and out they come.

"The principal way these various levels of disconnection manifest is fear, and principle amongst these is the fear of death, for which our traditional mechanisms are relatively absent in helping us to navigate. Yet any depth psychologist will tell you that the fear of death disguises the opposite; that is, an attraction toward it. I saw this in the circumstances surrounding Ann's death and came to see it many times in medical practice. It is vicarious, although it satisfies the imagination and indirectly faces what we all must, sooner or later.

"It is this deep fear that is embodied in pain and suffering: That we might die. But, instead of facing it and progressing through the redemptive trial of death-underworld-resurrection (or whatever alternative names you want to use for this process), it becomes a hurdle too big and we retreat from it in various psychological ways. Medicine sees this with all manner of trauma, illness and disease; it is as if there is a crossroads and the wrong path taken, with no turning back. And medicine can encourage this position with excessive focus on the problem, rather than uncovering what may be driving it. Instead, the agency of pain and suffering and its representation as a medical problem becomes the meaning with which to go on, until such time as death inevitably supervenes.

"Covid is the fear of death writ large on the collective stage and basically for the same reasons as within the individual. I recall when I started to notice the consequences of overuse of antibiotics and the subsequent rise of antibiotic-resistant bacteria, I foresaw that we may get into a similar fix with vaccination and viruses, even to predicting a decade or so ago that an infectious disease epidemic was quite likely, even inevitable. Social issues like overcrowding, city densities, nutritional and environmental concerns simply compounded this view. The arrogance of a medical profession that believes the tools at its disposal would counter any such event merely indicated to me that the profession itself had a greater fear than even the general public. After all, maybe this is what attracts people to become doctors in the first place.

"From a more internal perspective, we are metabolically imbalanced with nutritionally impoverished diets, generally unfit and overweight, and with little idea about how to support our immune systems, and with it our nervous and hormonal systems.

This is all hardly rocket science, but it has been pathetically overlooked by institutional medicine and its vested interests, who seem not to want the average individual to have the necessary information to rectify these imbalances and hence control of their own health destiny. Beneath any fear lurks a power dynamic of concerning proportion and intensity."

"Are you saying that such information is deliberately withheld?" I asked.

"I am not directly. But the lack of awareness is ignorance in the light of health and medical knowledge elsewhere, and its lack of integration into a more holistic and modern view is negligent at best and deliberately disempowering the public at worst. However, the information on how any person can actively support their immune and associated bodily systems, such as the old favourites of diet and exercise, is more accessible now.

"We could extend this information into more traditional and folk medicines, in areas like herbal medicine, and with these insights then approach the more shamanic and archetypal foundation of medicine. This is the holistic domain that pairs the physical with the psychological and reinforces a healthy and purposeful attitude, that itself leads into the whole area of mental health in modernity."

"How so?" I interjected.

"Well, firstly there is the mental stance that someone can take to support their general health, which is then a foundation for more specific attention to the immune system. Self-responsibility is a key factor, which goes a long way to balancing the expectation that others will tell you what to do, as well as the blame that can be associated with this. The inevitable outcome of not taking responsibility is seeing others as responsible, first for keeping you healthy, and second, as being responsible if you get ill.

"Supporting self-responsibility is empowerment. Power in

health is something we have touched on earlier, and I just want to reinforce how important it is, because it is readily understated and therefore 'given away' to others. We tend to have a negative view of power, readily reinforced by agencies and institutions that have more control over us, if we are rendered powerless. Power and control go together. Again, control is given negative connotations, as in 'control freak', but it is an important moderator and consequence of instinctual power. Power used consciously is empowerment; it does not use power as an agent for and exertion over another or others, in fact the opposite. This is one reason that I see the various institutions governing the pandemic as being relatively and concerningly powerless, because they need public acquiescence, instead of empowering people."

I found these insights challenging and could see how the dynamics of depth psychology could be used to explain what we may intuitively think, and also how the institutional position leads to polarization – not a good position to be in handling a pandemic. Nor generally in a supposed democratic world, I further considered. This naturally led into the whole area of political and social involvement in the pandemic.

"It is a little ironic that a supposedly democratic society behaves in such an authoritarian manner when something fearful arises. It is maybe cynical, but one view could be that it is an opportunity for more authoritarian control. The difference between our political system and more totalitarian ones may simply be that we use more coercion based on fear rather than absolute control. It could even be argued that the totalitarian systems are being less duplicitous and more honest."

I decided to let that one pass, as it may take us too far afield. But Kennan would have none of this. After a pause with no intervention on my part, he continued:

"The issues of social distancing, masks and vaccination

highlight my concerns in this whole area from the health perspective." Now he had my attention again.

"Social distancing is a poor term; physical distancing is more accurate. Using 'social' inverts the social connections that we so crave in times of threat and fear, giving them a negative connotation. That we need physical distancing, in the appropriate contexts at times of infectious disease, has long been known. So, shouldn't we just be simply educated, rather than have stipulations of 1.5 or 2m distancing mandated?

"Similarly with masks. In general, good education about infectivity and the value of mask-wearing in the appropriate circumstances would not be too difficult. As with physical distancing, there is enough fear to make most listen, and take the guidelines on board. But to mandate all people to wear masks at all times in designated circumstances is overkill and, I suspect makes little difference beyond good education. Conversely, it has a deleterious effect on the physical health of some vulnerable members of society, as well as having unrecognised and potentially more serious mental health problems. These can be long term and lead to more general fear in society; we have yet to see these consequences emerge, but emerge they no doubt will."

Here we were on common ground. Kennan was putting into context what I had suspected. As a society, we are already fearful, and these measures simply contribute further to the fear and stress. And we hadn't even got to the topic of vaccination, as yet: Kennan must have read my mind.

"Although medically trained, I have always had serious concerns about the use, effects and reach of vaccination in infectious disease, such that I question whether our modelling of such disease itself is in need of correction, even renewal."

A big statement; I trusted we would return to it and did not prompt Kennan, as he seemed on a roll.

"As a precursor, I need to say that I have progressively vaccinated less with my children. My last child had one tetanus jab only – and he reacted to that – and is now a healthy adult, although he will have had Covid jabs for his work. I am of the belief that many diseases of later life may be related to over-vaccination and lack of exposure to relatively mild illnesses in childhood."

"In general, I suspect we view vaccination for illnesses like viruses that don't respond to pharmaceutical chemicals, similarly to antibiotics for bacterial infections. And, as antibiotic usage becomes progressively problematic, even dangerous, I believe we will get into a similar mess with vaccinations, if we haven't already done so. Vaccination may have a significant place in the medical armoury, but its routine and widespread usage I have cause to question. We need to be more highly selective in where and how we use it, as well as to whom it is given. The apparent effectiveness of smallpox vaccination should not be used as a marker for all vaccinations, and even this is now coming into question.

"I also find it interesting that in spite of the common cold – itself a corona virus – defying all attempts to find a vaccine for as long as I can remember, we are almost immediately able to find several for Covid. There seem to be considerable vested interests here, certainly in the pharmaceutical industry and other associated business and political interests. Not only that, but we also have the opportunity to let loose a largely unknown vaccine that uses mRNA technology onto the general public; a relatively uncontrolled trial in my opinion, the concerns associated with using this for other genetic manipulation notwithstanding.

"It must be remembered that such epidemics have been around since time immemorial; they are part of life. Humans are afflicted by them in a wave-like manner over spans of years and have coped. Maybe the viruses themselves are a factor that improves our immune systems and has other more genetic effects presently unknown. That they also act as a culling mechanism for the old and infirm is relatively unfortunate in individual circumstances, but an inevitable part of life. Often, untreated respiratory illnesses are also nature's way of ending a life in a relatively gentle manner.

"You may argue that Covid is hardly peaceful, and certainly my own experience of SARS was not. But is this because we are distanced from these cycles and I, like others, have not had exposure to trivial problems like the common cold as often, or other infections that may serve a similar function? Are we vaccinating ourselves away from these forces in an attempt to allay the fears of all and preserve the lives of others who are somewhat compromised? These are difficult ethical questions, but medicine, here as in many other areas, tends to be attracted by advances and success at the expense of these deeper ethical questions.

"As a relative aside, it should not be forgotten that biological warfare is rife, in spite of various sanctions against it. There is a smoking gun behind Covid and its origins. If we are extending our poorly ethically controlled research and application in the genetic fields beyond what is acceptable – and I am sure that we are – then the virulence of pandemics may lack the normal checks and balances of so-called natural infections. And, by comparison, Covid may prove to be a relatively innocuous disease."

I squirmed in my seat a little.

"There are some other odd features with Covid. We see it as being infective, yet there is a strong vascular component that leads to lung and heart problems. It should not be forgotten that vaccination is also implicated in this area. This may be compounded by environmental factors, such as a sedentary lifestyle (think air flights and DVTs), lack of exercise, overcrowded city living, lack of exposure to nature and clean air. These are all, of course, components in the climate crisis that is at least partially caused by humanity's presence and actions, and conveniently somewhat obscured by Covid when these factors should instead be more highlighted.

"Yet we are simultaneously keeping the elderly alive, often longer than naturally, with the use of various pharmaceutical medications. Chief amongst these are drugs for high cholesterol and blood pressure. Somehow these seem to be fostering some of the vascular problems we are encountering in the lungs of those afflicted with Covid. Are such drugs a predisposition or even a trigger for severity and hence risk of infirmity and death? Also, many of the elderly on such medications are hardly living in socially conducive environments.

"I think I am getting into listing problems, rather than providing an appropriate argument here, Ian."

I agreed. There were other problematic issues that could be addressed, such as the role of 5G and others bordering on conspiracy theory maybe, but still not entirely put to rest. I was keener that, having created a platform of concern around Covid, Kennan would either provide alternatives or create a different platform. I was not to be disappointed.

"It may be worth considering that this current pandemic may not be an isolated event, but mark a succession of similar ones, or even a precursor of a more serious event to come. I base this feeling, albeit somewhat intuitive and prophetic, on the underlying trends and concerns in which the current pandemic should be more appropriately viewed."

"This concerns me more than a little, Kennan; your record of prophetic insights is good, so the fact that you see it this way is something that maybe I and others should listen to, even though I know that you are not alone. However, I would appreciate any insights that you may have that underpin this statement?"

"There are two main areas I would like to talk about. The first is prefaced by my comments a little earlier about climate change. That we are at least partially responsible for this, means that we are likely to see previously unknown or hidden problems emerge, such as different patterns of infectious disease; although how far man's hand is directly involved in these changes is difficult to gauge with any degree of certainty.

"So, almost in passing, I would like to stress that attending to climate change is a pre-requisite, but not only for dealing with infectious disease. The wider picture is that our environmental sensitivity needs to increase and there is evidence that this is occurring. One result of lock-downs and travel restrictions is that people are exploring more of their own immediate surrounds, as well as looking to see how they can unclutter and simplify their lives. I see these changes as alternatives that the pandemic has – seemingly incidentally – thrown up, although the mystic in me wonders about the hand of spirit here!"

We shared a quiet laugh here, as it was something I had noticed too and had wondered what may be driving such an increased sensibility. Such inversions are common, such as the increased perception of the value of our immediate family and social circles, whilst under the constraint of so-called 'social distancing'. I must admit that Kennan's reference to spirit's role may be accurate and our laughter a verbally mute recognition of this.

"Up until this point, we have seen Covid as the enemy; an enormous amount of power is being projected onto such a tiny being, indicating how much this is a psychological projection of our own powerlessness, including within the medical profession. The warfare mentality really is passé; not only with Covid, but with many illnesses and diseases, cancer most notably. Effectively, once infected, the virus is actually within us – part of us.

"So maybe we need to ask different questions, such as, what is its intention? With the exception of the elderly and the infirm, who may be in God's waiting room at the time of affliction, how may it be helping us? At the very least, this could be from an immunological point of point, as well as cleansing us of accumulated toxins. Also, viruses may have some sort of direct role on our genetic material, a kind of resetting or rebooting maybe?

"I don't think these are idle questions. I feel we should take them – and others that arise – very seriously. The view that we are all separate from each other and collectively from nature is really quite limited and restricted to a materialistic and strictly scientific worldview. We are interconnected and part of a relatively seamless whole, in my opinion, and this includes our view of nature as alive and nurturing; Lovelock's Gaia, in fact. If we continue to treat nature and her other inhabitants as the enemy, it is we – the human species – that may not survive. I believe we are finally getting this fundamental point; I just trust it is not too late."

After a reflective pause, I asked Kennan what his second point was.

"We may have the wrong view of infectious disease," was his response, "the view that it is to our detriment and should be treated in an adversarial manner is very limited and accurate only in certain circumstances. This view needs modifying, although to such a degree that it demands a paradigm shift in our thinking. Mind you, medicine as a whole needs such a kick up the arse, maybe Covid is just showing us the way.

"The view that we can somehow beat Covid with vaccination, masks, social distancing and drugs is limited and proving not to be the case; it is quite pathetic really and an insult to spiritual intelligence. The concession is that we are 'learning to live' with the virus, even though we don't accept it. In my view, this is an inevitable outcome, because it may be that the virus is not the actual cause of the disease, but only a factor in its genesis, or even a consequence of the infection. I am not alone in this view; something similar was proposed by Rudolf Steiner over a century ago."

I had heard of the mystic Steiner. He has had an enduring effect on society and culture, schools in his name are throughout the western world, and his biodynamics is an ecological and ethical approach to farming, gardening and nutrition that is fundamentally holistic. Essentially, Steiner saw the virus as being the consequence of the disease process, so if Kennan held similar views, I asked what the actual disease causation might be, if it were not the virus.

"The fact that some people don't get it points to factors that may have a genetic basis. Also, people who attend well to their immune systems are at least less severely affected. But overall, I guess one of the features of a paradigm shift in thinking about infectious disease is that these organisms do not cause the disease, but may be involved in it as a consequence of other factors.

"In the previous discussion, we talked about nature and our need to reconnect with her and all her kind in a fundamentally holistic way. I suspect that factors we have already talked about and are dotted throughout our discussions are involved in a matrix that can precipitate illness and disease. These are issues such as overpopulation, or specifically high density living. Disconnection from a natural lifestyle and our lives run by technology leads to stress, but also a spiritually-deprived existence.

"We are collectively overweight, unfit and nutritionally impoverished. Indeed, the poverty-stricken have inadequate diets, but for quite a different reason. We are also, in my opinion, over-vaccinated, and we treat all micro-organisms – even the ones that help and support us – as the enemy. We are over-sanitised, plaster ourselves and our environments with toxic material, and we somehow expect to remain well, or to have modern medicine do it for us.

"Infectious disease should not be primarily seen as a disease, but as a spectrum of our responses in our inter-relationship with the environment, specifically the micro-environment. Many of our modern diseases can be connected back to this estrangement from a dynamic, interconnected and holistic relationship with other creatures, the land, and existence at large. Our fear of death lumps all strangers into the predator category, including the ones we can't see, and probably because we have made our lifestyles relatively 'predator-less', then our imagination becomes paranoid and sees them where they don't exist.

"Maybe Covid at the existential level is indicating to us ways we can correct and rebalance our perspectives? If so, then it may be an agent in a disease process that may be helping us in ways that we can't as yet see. Maybe only time will tell, but it is worth tracking the disease and people who have been afflicted to see what outcomes may emerge.

"This is not to deny medical care to those that need it. But I do think that many of the measures around the way Covid is being managed are to protect an over-burdened and unnecessarily centralised health system and the science that supports it, backed up by technology and – God forsake us – data and statistics. In this medical model, fear is the enemy. So maybe the extension of what I am saying is that not only should we review our infectious disease model, but our medical model as a whole. If Covid is an agent in this process, it has done its job.

"In the greater scheme of things, society and culture must extend from and remain related to the forces that underpin its very existence. Modern medicine is nothing if it is not holistic, not just in its own jurisdiction, but also in the interconnected web of systems in which we are embedded. But we are not just restricted to this human-oriented web, there are also the other forces and energies on which we rest and which issues like climate change remind us of. If we forget this, we are at risk of being overwhelmed by these forces and become irrelevant. At some symbolic level, I believe this is what Covid is reminding us of.

"Maybe this is a collective Dark Night of the Soul for humanity to negotiate, like I and many others have done at the individual level. Having symbolically died, death does not hold the same significance for me. And this experience tells me that humanity must collectively face its own potential death, which it is otherwise attracting and even encouraging, otherwise this would not be a symbolic death and transition, but a literal death – that of our species. Because, irrespective, spirit will continue in its relentless pursuits with or without us."

Twenty

We are now looking at the horizon. Where can medicine go from here? What will it look like in the future? It has been fairly clear to me, all along the path Kennan and I have walked together, that he eschews an exclusively rational, scientific and technological foundation to this future. It is also clear that he has a sort of magical and teleological view of it. Should modern western medicine become more conscious of a lot of its deficiencies and blind alleys, Kennan feels it can be a major contributor to the changes and outcome. Should it not, it is in danger of being irrelevant, at least, or destructive to the creative process, at the very worst.

In Kennan's opinion, it requires MWM to see its own psychological 'shadow' in a collective and psychological sense. It needs to recognise what it has to offer moving forward, such as accident, emergency and trauma medicine, but also recognise those branches that aren't advancing and meeting the public need. It also needs to recognise its own psychology; because greed and arrogance, lack of empathy, disinterest, and generally issues of power and control are rife.

There are also the concerns about institutionalisation, which I know trouble Kennan greatly beyond his own experience of being on the receiving end, yet which the profession has adopted nonetheless. Maybe this is a rear-guard action by the perceived assailing forces, or maybe it is simply a collective phenomenon at large in western society: Irrespective, Kennan sees it as anachronistic and in need of restructuring. But with such political and institutional forces now firmly entrenched, he is not optimistic. Nor is he about the various governing bodies that permeate all levels of medical delivery, commonly without the necessary experience or insight.

Kennan's opinion is that change will come from the public as the recipients of healthcare, prior to the establishment changing its position. He sees that as already happening with the movement toward alternative and complementary medicine; although he is concerned about how the institutions are incorporating this change by stealth. He sees such forces as social media as important, though presently disorganised, as well as the cultural phenomenon of the new age movement to have a progressive input, as it matures and reaches into areas that MWM will not dare to.

So, I asked Kennan to give me his take. This would take the form of a soliloquy, I would discover, when I replayed the discussion and my notes. There were various points where I felt to intersect, but did not. I let him have his say and, with only some minor editing, I will present what he said verbatim.

"I am aware that by taking a strong traditional view to our contemporary malaises, I can be seen as regressive. But this is not an exclusive view. When we meet an impasse in the present, as I believe medicine is doing, then it is sometimes necessary to look to past patterns; not as historical and irrelevant, but as clues to things we may have lost sight of. Most particularly is the case with medicine. It is not to deny the advances, but when they are not meeting up to promised rewards, then maybe we need a revisioning process to be undertaken. I'm not alone in this opinion, and I would like to draw on the ideas of Carl Jung to give my argument both substance and a modern relevance.

"Jung developed something he called archetypal theory with more than a little philosophical influence, even stemming back to Plato. He saw an archetype a little like a prototype or a stereotype, if we need an analogy here. It is just that the word archetype has more of a mythic and symbolic relevance, which I hope will become apparent as I outline my viewpoint. By mythic I mean that an archetype has a timeless quality, in other words, it is always relevant. Archetypes tend to regulate their field of importance and do not take a dualistic or moral stance; that is, they just are and are neither right nor wrong.

"Medicine is an archetype. It describes the field of health and healing by elaborating its detail in patterns, sometimes in symbolic language, but also mythically. In other words, we can find these patterns in myth and sometimes in history, where it takes a more magical quality with distance from the present. It can be present in our stories, our ancestral history, and other sources. One of these sources can be other cultures that have preserved an unbroken line of tradition through history into prehistory, as well as recognising a common pattern across such different cultures.

"I would argue that MWM does not have that sort of continuity, as I hope I have illustrated in our discussions, with such cultural change as the Christian and Mediterranean usurpation of indigenous culture in Europe and the modern eruption of scientific rationality. I would also argue that the patterns in MWM are dissimilar to those of other cultures, where the similarities are more apparent than not. These patterns are present in the archaic tradition of shamanism, which is one revival that the new age movement has creatively contributed to.

"Another way to look at this is to distinguish two levels of reality; that is, the daily one of time and space, and the night-time one that is more mythic, creative, and imaginary, as we recognise in dreams. The Australian Aboriginal people have a specific name for this: The Dreamtime. Although other cultures, particularly the Meso-American, have a similarly differentiated view. But this is not just archaic, as modern quantum physics describes a similar twofold view of reality. You will have noticed in my account that, at various points, I felt I was dealing with quantum reality. A quantum medicine is premature, but could maybe define the medicine of the future, maybe through the arbiter of healing the mind-body split.

"Medicine is recognised in western culture as being the "science or art of diagnosis and treatment of disease". Yet I have issue with the word 'diagnosis', as it can literally mean 'to know apart'; that is, away from the person. As you know, I much prefer the word 'syndrome' or 'moving together'; where symptoms are collected into a unified whole in the person of the sufferer. It lends itself to the personal history, story, and extends to anecdote.

"Please note, once again, that the above definition gives medicine a pathological rather than a physiological definition. Medicine can also be something prepared or made for treatment or prevention, although today we commonly associate this term for medicine with pharmaceutical drugs, rather than herbs, foodstuffs or even salves and poultices.

"Yet there is another definition of medicine as a "spell, charm, or fetish believed to have healing, protective, or other power". This last definition has commonly been restricted to the North American Indian, but as I have and will continue to point out, it also has modern relevance, because it is part of the archetypal complex that is medicine.

"Many years ago, I developed a model for what the archetype of medicine would look like to modern eyes. It is relatively simple at one level, but leads into a depth if each of the paths is followed and elucidated, and which is where I would like to begin. We touched on this pattern earlier on, but here I want to give it more depth and context.

"Medicine can be broken down into four essential components, in my view. The dominant one in MWM is the scientific model of health. Yet this is just one health model amongst many. I have alluded to the humoural theory of our own history, from which we have become separated. This is the view that health is modelled around the so-called elements, bodily humours, and temperaments. This may sound quaint but, stemming from Culpeper in the early seventeenth century, this model still has current application amongst alternative medical practitioners.

"Of course, there are many more models, such as in Traditional Chinese or Ayurvedic Medicine, but the principle here is that we have a model of health. The problem here is that MWM, unlike most other models, has become almost exclusively centred around its scientific health principles, and ignored what I have nominated as the three other components.

"A second component is the medical practitioner or therapist. This is tacitly acknowledged in MWM, but is not given importance beyond being present to administer the protocol-ridden model. We have ignored the ritual of the consultation and treatment, as well as the power of the relationship itself. The ritual has become transferred, like the model of MWM itself, into pharmaceutical medicine and its delivery. The power is unacknowledged and often distorted as control, instead of using it to embrace the client or patient, so to empathise with and empower them in their own welfare. There is a connection here to the tradition of magic.

"Thirdly is the setting in which the treatment is conducted. I would suggest that the modern clinic is not very conducive to health and well-being. It is sterile, as are hospitals, literally, and not nurturing. What a contrast is a setting that employs nature, or allows animals, such as dogs and cats. Have we lost connection with the power of a retreat or even a pilgrimage? Why do places like Lourdes exist?

"These three components can all be seen to point to and

connect with the fourth component of healing. Medicine has reduced healing to curing, as in fixing, making the problem go away … healing is, by definition, more holistic. Healing implies well-being and not necessarily with a cure; a patient may have cancer and be well; dying can be a spiritual transition of healing. In our modern view, trauma becomes fixed and not healed, so it is no wonder we have problems with post-traumatic stress extending to stress generally. It is not difficult to see the mismanagement of trauma as the foundation of the disease process.

"Healing, in this viewpoint, can be seen to include the other components, yet also to transcend them by appreciation of the spiritual component. In this respect, healing has one foot in our day-to-day reality, but the other in mythic time or quantum reality."

"It may be useful to look at the shamanistic worldview to expand further on these points. Not only will this illustrate that shamanism is not a dead tradition, but it will also demonstrate how much of it adds depth and relevance to our modern medical worldview, and may contribute to its rejuvenation, even transformation. I would also point out that I am not taking the limited anthropological perspective of shamanism confined to Siberian culture, but an archetypal one that exists worldwide.

"In summary, the shamanistic worldview is as far back as you can go when looking for the roots and sources of health and medicine in humanity. I have found it rich and rewarding to explore, although I have tended to stay away from many of the new age interpretations, which I find often lack depth and real authenticity. This is partly because of the modern sensibility, which seeks to brand, authenticate, and promote health techniques in a manner that does not offend the western mentality. Shamanism defies such categorisation, in my opinion. Shamanism also encroaches on domains such as magic and power, as well as an acceptance of a worldview and reality that transcends our own; again, we are approaching a quantum physics worldview.

"This is an irony really: Einstein explored and charted this new territory that ventures into the shamanic worldview over a century ago. We still live in a Newtonian world, yet all around us are instruments such as lasers, the internet, and computers that stretch this to breaking point. But, in my view, it has already been superseded, because quantum physics indicates – although its proponents find difficulty in accepting – that the shamanic worldview of at least two apparently intersecting realities is how our existence is constructed. (Kennan stressed the word 'apparently', quite significantly.) If you have any grasp of the quantum world, you will see how it permeates the components of the shamanistic complex I am about to describe.

"We are accustomed to seeing the world around us as 'inorganic' or lacking in life. Not only does the quantum worldview negate this, but also shamanism exists in an animated world. Animism is not simply a primitive form of religion – assuming monotheism is somehow an advance on this – but it is the background to a polytheistic worldview that shapes our imaginations, creativity, and myths.

"In practical terms, how does this affect MWM? Well, shamanism sees infection as animated and purposeful, as well as diseases like cancer having a meaning beyond the limited manner that we see it. It sees trauma as not just a psychological event, but woven into our history, even beyond the personal to the ancestral. It understands mental distress as visitation of energetic patterns (maybe recognised as entities) that may create a schism within us, called soul loss, making us susceptible to visitation of illness and disease.

"In further practical terms, we can see this in stress making us susceptible to a common cold, or even the beginnings of cancer. We can see visitation as responsible for conditions like schizophrenia and mania, when there is metaphorically 'nobody home' or 'being out of their mind'. We can appreciate that the modern phenomenon of UFOs might be an interpretation of something ancient, like elves and dwarves, or even the 'gods'. Even paranoia can extend into this realm and be a psychological reflection of its very existence, if we remain 'open-minded' enough – yet another metaphor.

"What extends from this view of life is something remarkable. The scientific perspective has tended to form a seemingly impermeable boundary around its own worldview, calling anything outside 'mystical', 'imaginary' or 'childish', in a demeaning and deprecatory way. Yet, ironically, it is science itself that is wrestling with the boundary between the daily and mythic realities; not only in quantum physics, but in chaos theory, string theory, imaginary numbers in mathematics, and such practical application as lasers and other tools of medical technology that rely on the quantum perspective. Even neuroscience, supposedly at the forefront of research of the mind, struggles with this straitjacket.

"Shamanism sees the boundary as permeable. It recognises that there are people who can live a marginal existence with one step in each, which psychiatry – a medical discipline itself under severe question – has tended to call schizophrenic, bipolar, or epileptic. But there is a qualitative difference between those who can travel in these strange worlds and those who cannot thrive in it; the former is the shaman, the latter the madman.

"What makes the difference? Essentially, the shaman has commonly experienced an illness that may be life-threatening, as well as having serious psychological effects – if there ever is this lack of relationship – and who emerges from the experience with the wisdom and guidance of a mentor, already having trodden the path. This is basically seeing illness and disease as an initiation. Most particularly in the psychological realm do we see the consequences of this process being aborted, where psychiatry blocks it with drugs and social policing, and reinforced socially, from family to society. We may be drugging our mystics and prophets and then calling them madmen and women.

"The extension of this is that the shaman sees ritual and initiation to be essential parts of life. Is this why we have troubled youth, because they do not have a rite of passage into adulthood? Are they using drugs to attempt a broadened perspective of life, and not to just get high? Is the fact that these drugs are now no longer botanical, but refined chemicals, the reason they become addicted? And why should we be surprised, when we teach them in their upbringing that there is a pill for every ill, even though there is a deep and paradoxical truth in this manoeuvre? Yet we simultaneously ban them from using botanical agents that have been used from time immemorial to explore life's mysteries: Who is actually mad in this worldview?

"The shaman is the person in the tribe or culture who conducts the rituals for the community, as well as for individual or collective healing. There is an understanding of nature, the skies and the underworld to facilitate these at the correct time of the day, month, or year, depending on the purpose and specifically so for healing. But how does the shaman learn this; is it simply by being mentored? Whilst this may be the case, it is because – by definition – the shaman is the 'master of ecstasy'. (Please note that, although I am using the male gender here by custom, the terms refer to both sexes.) What this means is that the shaman, by virtue of his or her marginal existence, is able to travel between the worlds. How is this performed?

"The shaman enters an altered state of consciousness, guided by a ritual or ceremonial structure. There is often the assistance of a rhythmic beat, through a drum or rattles, which are known to affect the electrical pattern of the brain pattern and alter it. Also, other specific techniques can be used, such as the sensory deprivation and heat of a sweat lodge ceremony, or fasting. Of course, the use of drugs has reached the popular imagination here, and not always in a good light. This was and is not universal, and if it is then botanical hallucinogens are used, and generally in a ritual context.

"It is customary to use assistance for this travelling. Commonly this is by or with what is known as a 'power animal', that is of the shaman's preference. The shaman takes on the identity of the animal, which is quite feasible with an animistic worldview, and which the shaman experiences as literal and not simply imaginary. Even those around him or her may witness the animal and not the human form. But where does the shaman go? According to the outline I've given, it is into mythic or quantum reality. At one level this can be seen to be the imagination. But is that all it is? The shaman would say it is real, that he or she actually is in the other reality, or the dreamtime, if you will.

"What is done there? Here we enter a world that is hardly conventionally psychiatric. The shaman may have a task to fulfill for the community, but it is often associated with healing, and is employed specifically so for individual cases. Commonly this takes the form of soul retrieval. The theory is that the illness or disease is because part of the soul may be split off by stress or trauma and disconnected from the individual, and the shaman's task is to retrieve it and bring it back into the afflicted person. The reverse of this is also true: a deranged person may have an invasion of a force or entity that has possessed them, commonly because the soul is lost, and in such a situation shamanic exorcism is also employed.

"If you think I am in a fantasy world with what I am explaining, then ask any good psychotherapist about their work, because it is what they do if they venture beyond the cognitive realms. They may not see it as such, and in the modern context the therapist is often assisting their clients to do their own mental journeying or psychic travelling to heal themselves, but the principle is the same.

"But this is not just for mental disturbance. As I pointed out earlier and a holistic worldview substantiates, mental disturbance is seen as a factor in all illness and disease, including the physical. In fact, and shamanism would argue this, physical illness stems from mental, emotional, and ultimately spiritual disturbance, and not the other way around. I would agree with this, even if only that the orientation should be psychological toward the physical and not the reverse. The perennial philosophy also would agree here."

"What the shamanic worldview engages, directly or indirectly, is healing. It takes the health component of my earlier modeling into the healing one. If you look at my fourfold model, you can also see that shamanism engages all of the components much more fully than MWM. However, there are some loose ends that can maybe flesh out this perspective a little further.

"I have tried, wherever possible, to show how the shamanistic perspective is not regressive or archaic, but links to or underpins the modern worldview. This can be explored in much more detail, and is a necessary ongoing inquiry, in my opinion. What I am trying to illustrate is that it satisfies the archetypal perspective of medicine far better than MWM does presently, which is why I use it, and is also why many alternative and complementary practitioners do partially or completely, in one form or another.

"Actually, the shamanic term for the healer is a 'medicine man (or woman)'. Healing exists within the overall shamanic complex, although a shaman is not necessarily a medicine man, even though the functions overlap considerably. The shaman can take on more of a priestly function, or be primarily a magician. In many ways, the mythic figure of Merlin, and his modern recreation as Tolkien's Gandalf, fits the magical aspect, although it could be seen that both have a healing function, even if only at the community level.

"This is the aspect of the healing definition, where "a spell, charm, or fetish believed to have healing, protective, or other power" comes in. This is the healer as magician, who can negotiate mythic reality with soul retrieval, and uses a ritual for the purpose. Charms are still commonly used, and a spell is employed to imbue them with the power of words, often poetic, for healing or magic. A fetish is simply an object or talisman that can be worshipped because it is imbued by magical power, which may be evoked by the shaman.

"What can be seen from this is the extraordinary intensity that exists between the medicine man and his or her patient. Modern hypnosis employs the use of the word in a ritual structure, not unlike the medicine man. Also, the emotional intensity of the therapeutic relationship, including its erotic nature, can be employed for healing, as well as being more magically used for divination and prophesy.

"Personally, I do not find it difficult to context MWM in this overall broader, deeper, more archetypal worldview. I find it enriching and informative. It also highlights the deficiencies of modern medicine and where to look for retrieval of the lost components and even the art itself. It is certainly rewarding to use in healing settings like the workshop and retreat in ritual or ceremonial expression.

"At the core of this view, though, is the notion of power. Without power, there is no healing, no magic. The physicians of the past knew how to employ this for the benefit of their patients; they were not stripped of it by a well-meaning (maybe) institutional overview in the supposed public safety interests. It touches on the magical, but the recognition by the shaman is that this power is not his or hers, but something they 'tap into' in mythic reality and use for man's benefit and healing.

"It may be useful to now refer to the great chain of being and to see it as a link between the shaman's worldview and that of modern medicine. One of my major criticisms of the modern era is that we take what I call a bottom-up approach to reality. So, we start with the physical and then approach the emotional, mental and spiritual with the tools that we use for the physical domain. I think this is where psychiatry, neuroscience, and academic or research psychology get themselves into difficulty.

"If we take the converse, a top-down approach, then we can see the physical in a more inclusive manner as the shaman does, and not get into a lot of the cognitive difficulties that we do. Also, this approach sees the two realities of the non-physical – metaphysical – and physical in some sort of continuum, with a boundary between, sure, but a more available and permeable one. The shaman lives at this boundary and is why he or she is referred to as leading a liminal or marginal existence, knowing the keys to the portals of any permeable boundary.

"I think this perspective, together with the shamanic or archetypal reality, offers much to medicine, particularly the current difficulties with mental health that neuroscience may be exploring, but not solving. We commonly see the mental realms in a metaphoric way, such that 'he is out of his mind', or 'I don't know what possessed her'. Also, what we refer to as neurotic issues tend to be better seen in the context of fear, insecurity, loss of faith, direction, purpose and meaning.

"Modern psychology has made inroads, but these are limited. Approaches like cognitive behavioural therapy (CBT) are adaptive, but not healing. The depth psychological direction, started in the Freudian era, has extended further into the mental domains, uncovering the role of sexuality in health and illness.

This has been taken appreciably further by people like Jung, who explored mystical approaches like alchemy to discover the roots of health and healing in the spiritual domains.

"Then there are disciplines in modern medicine that have sought a more integrative approach. For example, psycho-neuroimmunology sees the psyche (mind or soul), brain, hormonal, and immunological systems as intimately interconnected, including the more fundamental axis between mind and body. There is a kind of fluidity to these bodily systems that makes them poorly responsive to the purely mechanical approaches of physical medicine and, placed together, they necessitate a holistic perspective.

"Even when we look at the purely physical domain, we ask deeper questions. Why was I vulnerable to getting this cold? What made me trip and break my leg? We even use metaphors such as "I was asking for that!" and see the body symbolically, as in "what is my low back pain expressing ... lack of support?" As an exercise, it is intriguing to make lists like these; it is fun to do at a workshop!

"Ultimately, though, we are approaching a holistic view, as I espoused earlier. Not only do we take account of the body and mind in a more integrated way, but also, we see our role in the world – occupational, family, environmental, and social – to be reflections of this. In the shamanic worldview, there is no separation. Recall that the shaman who shapeshifts to a power animal is not just imaging this; he or she actually becomes and is the animal!

"Yet we do not need to stop here. The plethora of eastern and new age approaches seem to carry truth at different levels, and for different practitioners. Also, as I have pointed out, the public is seeking these alternatives over MWM in a progressive manner. It is important that we look at the wisdom each carries. Even crystals and reiki have a place, if only in faith and their magical application; although myth tells us more that we have yet to discover, even with these apparent new-age approaches.

"But I am most interested in the heritage of my own culture. In this, I follow Jung. He explored western alchemy in depth and saw its modern relevance. We would do well to return chemistry and hence pharmacy to these traditional roots when applied to healing – at least. Alchemy is also a technique that has been used in healing and spiritual development from the dawn of time, and the alchemist is a more recent historical version of the shaman in the west.

"My own interest is in the Celtic and Anglo-Saxon traditions. I consider there is much wisdom that can be applied from these to the restoration of the medical archetype, and this ancestral heritage may speak to us in ways that other traditions do not. Many question Christianity for this simple reason, and are now looking to their heritage for spiritual direction. In my opinion, the veneer is much thinner than we think, the folk traditions lie close to the surface in the things we do, as well as say, such as in a charm to accompany it – 'touch wood'!

"It is rather a large leap to see the relevance and significance of the Anglo-Celtic traditions to modern medicine, so I will need to create some bridges for people to follow my argument. One of these would be to scratch the modern veneer and reveal how we still employ such things as alternative medicinal approaches based on faith; use fetishes, as well as employ charms and spells in health and well-being. I would explore this further by illustrating how, in our use of language, we retain many metaphors from our past and use rituals more extensively than we commonly appreciate.

"I would use Greco-Roman humoural medicine and people like Culpeper and Paracelsus as a bridge to the past and a more holistic perspective, where the mind and body are seen as a continuum. But I would also step outside of medicine into medieval literature to see in our myths, legends, and art the ongoing influence of fields like magic and healing, and a further bridge to a past that sits in the hinterland beyond history into myth.

"I find all this fascinating and exciting. It is also where my future lies …

"Yet there is one profound difference between archaic and modern shamanism, and this is the whole field of consciousness. I have avoided bringing in this terminology to date in the present discussion because it means so many things to different people. But I don't think I can avoid it now! I know we discussed this a lot earlier in our earlier meetings, relative to psychology and psychiatry, but I would like to pick up on that theme with respect more to the field of consciousness itself, within which shamanism is embedded.

"In the modern era, we have an individualised sense of consciousness that probably was not present to the same extent in times past. The way that this translated then was that the medicine man did the healing for the patient and the shaman conducted the ceremonies for the community. But now, the onus is more on the individual to conduct their own healing and develop their own spiritual practice.

"I think I sort of hinted at this with the role of the modern psychotherapist who operates beyond the mechanistic view of the mind, where he or she helps the client develop their own insight into their problems, blockages, or trauma. From here he or she can mentor the healing pathway with instruction, guidance, and support. This is a different emphasis from the shaman of old; the modern psychotherapist is directly empowering the client.

"I believe the imperative is for us collectively to make a connection with this deeper reality, not just in health and medicine, which itself may simply be in a similar sorry state to many establishments and professions. I think that is why the word 'unconscious' was so widely used in the recent past for this reality, but to me is a problematic term when it is more like 'expanded consciousness', 'awareness' or the like. That's why I try and avoid using such terms because they describe the phenomenon from the position it is looked at from, when there simply is no clear objective perspective.

"Ultimately, it comes down to the individual with all his or her subjectivity. We all need to take individual responsibility for our health, prior to and maybe as well as engaging others. We need to be empowered, or see only professionals who would empower us. In effect, we need to be in control of our own health and well-being as a wellspring of our destiny. We need to apply our own subjectivity and temper it by feeling, rather than looking outside for objective truth. Symptoms, physical or mental, tell us something is wrong. And they tell us directly; they don't text the doctor; so first and foremost, they represent health information, to and for us. We can be more educated in this, and use professionals who assist this process, not ones who would demean our attempts in this direction.

"We need to have some sort of reflective, contemplative, or meditative process in place. Here we can focus creatively and imaginatively on our health concerns that may, after all, be metaphoric and symbolic. And we can use that language – it is a capacity we all have, rather like intuition – it, maybe, needs some work and training. A journal is a simple and good place for us all to start. Here we can at least listen to our deeper intuitive lives within the greater spiritual reality by recording our dreams. They are symbolic and, symbolism if listened to, has a healing effect without needing to rationally understand it. We can also encourage this relationship by writing personal reflections, both to our dreams, but also to life concerns generally. It can also be a place to exercise our creativity; another function that bridges realities.

"Above all, we need to engage professionals who would inform, guide, and mentor us in this endeavor. Should we take that responsibility and inform our doctors, they may be relieved of the burden and help us in that process. If they don't, they are not for us. The power dynamic is shifting in the medical profession; it is no longer the doctor who wields the power in the therapeutic relationship, it is you, the patient-cum-client. Then into this mix we can add, as a component, all that MWM has discovered, learned and achieved."

We again, and for the last time in this context, stood and hugged in silence, then went home.

Epilogue

Ian Cook

How would I summarise Kennan's position – now mine – with respect to Modern Western Medicine? It's taken me a while, but I think I have found a way. Far from being a falsehood, as in the modern vernacular, a myth can be seen as something truer than truth. This may be seen as a paradox or an inversion of current logic, but nonetheless it rings true to me. So, what is the myth of modern medicine?

Maybe it is technology. And medicine is governed by technology. There is also a difference between technique, as art, and technology, as science. Medicine is no longer humanistic, and it is both distant from and opposite to healing. Technology is driven by science, which now defines medicine with its statistical so-called evidence-based medicine and pharmaceutical control. Doctors are technicians, deliverers of protocols, and dispensers of drugs.

The myth of technology is self-servicing, circular, and dehumanising when it comes to medicine, at least. If it ever gets out of its obsession with materialism it is only in a cognitive way. There is no entrance room for anything apparently less substantial, particularly if it contravenes the laws of science and technology. Other myths are dealt with by exclusion, derision, and metaphoric murder, particularly if they directly challenge or compete with the prevailing myth.

It is an irony that this modern myth only captures the cognitive aspects of the mind, as these are the only ones that support it. Anything else in the realm of mind – not to mention emotion, soul, or spirit – is either reduced to the cognitive or rejected by exclusion and derision (yet again). Not only that, but the 'gods' that govern other myths do not show their faces to those who are disbelieving and closed in their thinking.

We are left with a medicine that is mechanical. It sees the causes of illness and disease to be only in the realms it understands. This may be fine if you break your leg or are at the wrong end of a road accident. It may help to get over the hump of a cardiac arrest or overwhelming pneumonia. But, even after that hump, the question should be: "What got me into this mess in the first place?" And here we still only look mechanically.

Not only does Kennan see that the myth of medicine and its archetypal expression needs renewing and expanding, he also sees that such a viewpoint must include an expanded, creative and even artistic view of the apparent causes of illness and disease. In this more mythic position, he sees that trauma is unavoidable and indispensable to our personal and spiritual evolution, also that we need to see stress in a more creative and wholesome manner. Human existence is stressful. Period. We need to learn how to use it creatively, to negotiate trauma – including disease – in a meaningful and purposeful manner.

Kennan also sees that we must include everything in medicine. Science has the habit of excluding facts that do not fit the theory, which then becomes preordained. The placebo effect needs inclusion: Why do people recover – spontaneously – from potentially fatal diseases? What do these people do that is different? What is their story, their experience? The progression of medicine is littered with unusual discoveries from chance and haphazard events, now excluded from the scientific gaze. Maybe we need to reinstate the priests and philosophers of the medical art.

I also know that Kennan has a fundamental belief: that if we explore all the facts and stories that modern medicine excludes – because they don't fit – then we would end up with a very different medicine to the one we now have. Deep down, at the core, this is why Kennan left practice; he felt he wanted to explore, express, and work in this neglected territory. He was drawn into medicine exactly because of this brute fact; it had just taken several decades to realise that was his role and contribution. And this is what the present book is: A detailed preface to that adventure!

We don't need more doctors, drugs, and technology. We need more medicine men and women who understand the non-physical realms of health and disease and can negotiate it. We need elders and mentors who can support and guide us through our traumas and diseases; be that to renewed life, or death. We need such guides to alleviate our fears around pain, infirmity, and disease, so they do not dictate to us and define us to a lifeless life. We need a medicine that is optimistic, vital, and integrated into the whole of our life.

Maybe a final visionary quote from Kennan is appropriate:

"The future of medicine exists in the margins between fact and fiction; matter and energy; spirit and body, and a genuine 'psychogenetics' inclusive of myth, heritage, ancestry, and physical genetics. The art of the doctor is in living within this liminal state, and manipulating it for the welfare of patient, family, society and culture. To do this, he or she must enter the world of the soul and explore the poetry, magic, and sexuality that lies at the core of human transformation, and is the root of healing."

Afterword

Kennan Taylor

Following Ian's death in 2021, maybe there needs to be an 'afterword' on my part, as events have moved rapidly in this intervening period to the completion of this account, a year later. This will be a kind of stand-alone section, as the input of Ian's about me in the later chapters are very much his understanding of what was emerging for me during 2019 and subsequently since.

It was at this time that the cancer that would eventually take Ian's life some two years later was first diagnosed, although it was a somewhat predictable outcome of a long-term illness, that had also provided the common ground for us to work together and write this account in the first place. It also marked the end of our formal meetings, so this afterword is about occasionally correcting and clarifying some parts of the latter chapters provided by Ian, as well as recounting how things have moved on after his death in 2021.

It would be appreciated that in preparing for his passing, Ian's emphasis around this account would have taken on a different tone. Indeed, there were times where the cohesion between us was tested, although he was determined to finalise our project as best he could, for which I am truly grateful.

Even though not in my hands now, I continued to return to Ganieda to perform a ceremony and a sweat lodge ritual on specific seasonal and other occasions, for our small spiritual community in Albany that had gathered over the years. Some months after Ian's death, I returned for one such weekend to find that Ganieda, which I had passed back into the Bank's possession over a year before, was being purchased by an old chiropractic colleague. He had lost his own property, also being developed as a retreat elsewhere in the Albany region with the end of his marriage, and had then bought Ganieda as a 'going concern'. He approached me, asking for my involvement in the ongoing vision for Ganieda, with which he found compatibility and wished to combine into his own with my input. The old spiritual adage of losing everything to gain what you want came to mind; but I won't wax too lyrical. I just felt immense gratitude and respect for the man's open-hearted and generous offer.

This rather surprising turn of events has allowed me time to consolidate what Ian expressed earlier into a more tangible framework, as Ian's perspective tended to stress the teaching components – reflecting his own interests – whereas mine were gravitating more to other more psychospiritual areas, though still inclusive of some teaching. My work has settled into a more ritual and ceremonial framework, with teaching and healing practice around this. I continue with a clientele, mostly distant and online, whilst working on further teaching and training outlines. Creativity, fostered in my time in the den, is now an essential part of my life, even the backbone. In addition to completing this rather stuttering account, I have written a sequel to my rune book of nearly a decade before and am presently completing a work on the Grail legends. I see myself as a polymath and wordsmith.

After all the trials and tribulations of my career, I feel I have finally come home. I see that I have matured into some sort of eldership position within the community, where healing, teaching and training, and mentorship work are married to my creativity. Life is good, but it is always subject to change!

Although writing this section has revealed to me how much I still miss my friend ...

Postscript

Well, I'm done; I don't think I have any more to say about medicine … in its modern incarnation, that is. I have a lot to say about medicine in other incarnations, and how it will look in the future. But that's the stuff of, as yet, unwritten accounts.

As I read and reflect on the above narrative, I wonder whether I'm just pissing into the wind. Realistically, I'm not sure how many would want to listen to the stories and my interpretations of them, unless they knew me. But there is an imperative within me that has made me go through with this venture; maybe simply so I can move on.

I have this urge to put this narrative in another context now. I don't want to spend the rest of my life arguing with or trying to persuade others about the flaws in modern western medicine and what they need to do about it. You either 'get it' or you don't. I have done my bit, or duty if you will, to help you get it.

It is going to be comparatively easy for those who want to criticise me and this work as subjective, reactive, anecdotal, irrational and the like. Also, I realise I would be the subject of all sorts of psychological accusations, rather like Ian tried in the early days, as well as the stories being the subject of so-called fact-checking. I hope that makes anyone so inclined feel better. Seriously. But if you can, do better …

I feel that it has got to the time where the individual needs to – must – learn about home or folk medicine: How to cater for his or her own needs and those around them; then to look to how the community can support them – and vice versa, and which professionals to choose … and why?

Into the future, this may be a necessary foundation for a wholesome existence. I actually believe, if we are to survive as a species, that it is the people who listen to and enact this injunction are the ones who will set the tone for the future.

And it is these – in embryo presently, maybe – to whom this book is directed. Those who would take responsibility, be empowered, and undertake self-management of health as a foundation.

But this appeal is not simply directed at personal survival. It is directed toward the cultural and spiritual rejuvenation that we all need, even as a species.

Blessed be.

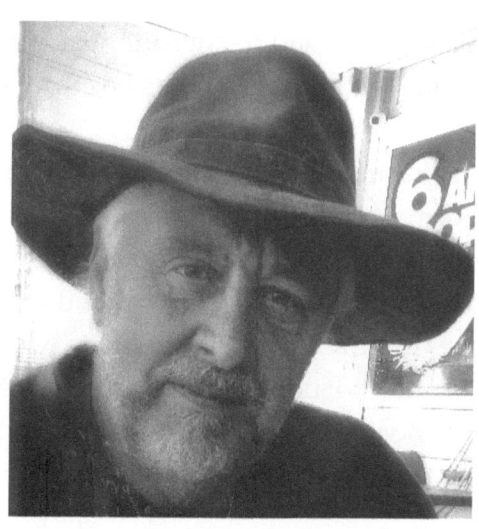

About the Author

My work is with the recovery and reinstatement of the soul, individually and within our modern culture. By my degrees, qualification and experience, I am an Oxford and London trained physiologist and medical doctor; by training and former practice a Jungian analyst; by initiation a Druid and shamanic healer; by decree an ordained priest and an elder in my tradition, and by disposition an alchemist, poet and wordsmith.

My former work as a general practitioner, holistic physician, and medical psychotherapist has been a preparation for this present path.

I am called to wrest from obscurity the ground between a dying religion, and a soul-less science ….

Volumes of knowledge and experience to be shared and dispensed to those who ask, and would listen.

An alchemist's robe I wrap around an ageing frame, a magical staff to feel my way, my heart beating to an ancient tune. A poetic sensibility is my torch.

A call to healing, vision and re-enchantment, a social cohesion of life-minded souls, a community to lead us through the darkest of times.

My heritage is in the northern spiritual traditions, specifically druidry, shamanism, and alchemy.

I bring these into modernity through the agencies and disciplines of medicine, depth psychology, and magic.

My landscape is now Australia; working with people and culture to forge a new identity and direction; clarifying meaning and purpose; grounded in ritual and ceremony, and the offerings that unfold; a direction encapsulated in the beating heart.

Contact details: drkennan1@gmail.com

www.ingramcontent.com/pod-product-compliance
Lightning Source LLC
Chambersburg PA
CBHW030049100526
44591CB00008B/79